Your First Year

—With—

DIABETES

What to do, month by month

Written and Illustrated by
THERESA GARNERO, APRN, BC-ADM, MSN, CDE

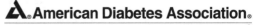

Cure • Care • Commitment®

Director, Book Publishing, Robert Anthony; *Managing Editor, Book Publishing,* Abe Ogden; *Editor,* Greg Guthrie; *Production Manager,* Melissa Sprott; *Composition,* ADA; *Illustrations,* Theresa Garnero; *Cover Design,* pixiedesign, llc; *Printer,* Transcontinental Printing.

Printed in Canada
1 3 5 7 9 10 8 6 4 2

The suggestions and information contained in this publication are generally consistent with the *Clinical Practice Recommendations* and other policies of the American Diabetes Association, but they do not represent the policy or position of the Association or any of its boards or committees. Reasonable steps have been taken to ensure the accuracy of the information presented. However, the American Diabetes Association cannot ensure the safety or efficacy of any product or service described in this publication. Individuals are advised to consult a physician or other appropriate health care professional before undertaking any diet or exercise program or taking any medication referred to in this publication. Professionals must use and apply their own professional judgment, experience, and training and should not rely solely on the information contained in this publication before prescribing any diet, exercise, or medication. The American Diabetes Association—its officers, directors, employees, volunteers, and members—assumes no responsibility or liability for personal or other injury, loss, or damage that may result from the suggestions or information in this publication.

♾ The paper in this publication meets the requirements of the ANSI Standard Z39.48-1992 (permanence of paper).

ADA titles may be purchased for business or promotional use or for special sales. To purchase this book in large quantities, or for custom editions of this book with your logo, contact Jewelyn Morris, Special Sales & Promotions, at the address below, or at JMorris@diabetes.org or 703-299-2085.

American Diabetes Association
1701 North Beauregard Street
Alexandria, Virginia 22311

Library of Congress Cataloging-in-Publication Data

Garnero, Theresa.
  Your first year with diabetes / Theresa Garnero.
      p. cm.
  Includes bibliographical references and index.
  ISBN 978-1-58040-301-6 (alk. paper)
  1. Diabetes--Popular works. I. Title.

  RC660.4.G366 2008
  616.4′62--dc22

                                2008016634

To all of the people who are living with or affected by diabetes.

Thanks to everyone who taught me about diabetes,
to Rosie Castillo for her relentless encouragement,
to my supportive colleagues, and
to the American Diabetes Association
for entertaining the notion of a very different book.

CONTENTS

Introduction

Diabetes is about change—changing your life from the way it was and bringing changes to your mind, body, and spirit. You *can* affect this disease and make changes in your favor, especially if you equip yourself with the latest resources contained throughout this interactive book. Every day, every hour, every minute presents an opportunity to make decisions that affect your health and well-being.

Diabetes is a balancing act and much more than a numbers game. It is a disease that requires paying attention to detail, while trying to maintain a positive attitude. The synergy of the mind-body connection is the key to long-term success in dealing with the disease. The more you participate and take things in stride, the better prepared you will be to take care of your health. And despite your best effort, diabetes management is demanding and rarely predictable. You will have slip-ups. You will have successes. Be your own champion.

Diabetes can also be overwhelming. This book provides you with easy-to-digest information you can use through the next year. One size does not fit all. Each person is unique. That's why you are given many options. *You* decide what to incorporate and what may work for your specific situation.

You will also likely learn that diabetes is a powerful motivator for health. It is my honor to be remotely involved with your journey and to share my unique perspective as a certified diabetes educator who has firsthand knowledge of the behind-the-scenes research and, equally as important, has experience with the real-life situations shared with me by thousands of people and their families dealing with diabetes. The result of this repository of evidence is a hands-on book with a positive approach to managing diabetes.

You'll read about the science of diabetes throughout these pages. You'll find health icons for easy navigation, light-hearted humor, and exercises that allow you to reflect on your progress. The art is in how you apply it to your everyday life. Diabetes requires paying attention to your health. It is not a death sentence, just a sign of mortality. This book is designed to help you make a connection with what works for you, find what is meaningful, and thrive in your life and in the passion that keeps you going. Let's get started!

How to Use this Book

Throughout this book, you'll notice icons. These are the interactive keys to diabetes self-care behaviors and will help you navigate this book and your diabetes. You can easily identify a self-care behavior based on the symbols. At the end of each section, choose *one* item to focus on or write in your own. Health outcomes or benefits happen by making small changes over time. And it's never too late to start.

Symbol	Related Key to Diabetes Self-Management
	Eat wisely
	Be active
	Check numbers (includes glucose/A1C, blood pressure, cholesterol, and weight)
	Reduce stress
	Understand medications
	Avoid problems
	Reduce risks
	Add humor

Adapted from the AADE 7™ Self-Care Behaviors.

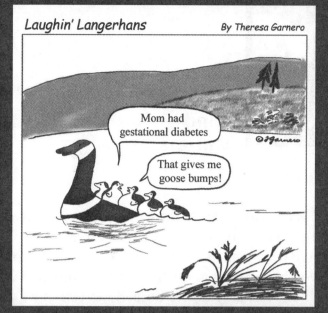

Week 1

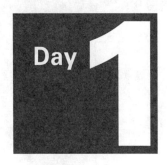

Day 1

Mind Matters

I was told I might have diabetes — *now* what?
Take a deep breath. Preparing your mind for your journey with diabetes is one of the best first steps to take. Being told you have diabetes, or that there is a problem with your blood sugar level, or that you are "borderline" can cause quite a bit of stress—and rightly so.

Diabetes is scary. You may have read headlines about what can go wrong or witnessed firsthand the negative effects of uncontrolled diabetes. Maybe you have been in denial that anything is wrong. That's OK. Denial protects and buffers you from difficult or shocking information. Do you feel guilty? Like you caused diabetes? If so, your first assignment is to stop the blame game and get on your own side. Anger, too, is a common reaction and is often the first sign that you acknowledge that something is wrong. It is never too late to jumpstart your diabetes self-management program. The key is to be gentle with yourself because you are your best resource for managing your diabetes.

Diabetes is never convenient, but with some effort and help from the experts, it *is* manageable. It is important that you acknowledge this. How you perceive this diagnosis will greatly impact the level of success with which your diabetes is managed.

The mind-body connection is real. Your thoughts and feelings have an enormous impact on the body. Positive thoughts have positive physiologic repercussions in the body, which is why humor is sprinkled throughout these pages. Humor is a useful tool in helping manage diabetes by adding perspective—not that there is anything funny about having diabetes. But a little humor may help you see from a different perspective. Humor can help you build the confidence to know that you *can* deal with diabetes. Plus, laughing lowers glucose levels!

Let's focus on something positive about your diabetes diagnosis. Feel free to say the following out loud:

- "I can follow my dreams and passions."
- "Diabetes sucks, but I can manage it."
- "I am not alone. Millions of people are dealing with diabetes and thousands of health care professionals are fighting to make a difference in my life and the lives of others."
- "The feelings I have about diabetes—be it anger, depression, fear, eagerness to learn, or relief at finding out—are typical. I have the strength to do something about my diabetes."

Diabetes does not define you; it's just a small part of your complex being. When it comes to diabetes, your treatment plan starts with being mentally prepared. What are some ways you are willing to deal with the stress of your diabetes diagnosis?

PERSONAL GOAL

Today (date _____), I decided I can (*check one*):

- ☐ Acknowledge how I feel about my diagnosis.
- ☐ Take a time out: see a movie, go for a scenic drive, or meditate.
- ☐ Listen to a favorite piece of music.
- ☐ Start a journal.
- ☐ Enjoy a bubble bath.
- ☐ Visualize my favorite vacation destination for 5 minutes.
- ☐ Stop negative self-talk.
- ☐ Look for a silver lining.
- ☐ Plan for problems (in both daily life and life with diabetes).
- ☐ Other: _____.

The good news is that I am coping. The bad news is that I maxed out my credit card!

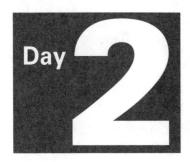

Day 2

Diagnosis: Diabetes

What is diabetes?

People often refer to diabetes as "a touch of sugar." This statement is an oversimplification. Diabetes is the end result of a complex, hormonal issue that relates to the body's ability to make and use insulin and get energy from foods.

All food is eventually converted into glucose (the technical name for sugar). Our bodies have millions of microscopic cells that use glucose for energy. The pancreas, a gland located behind the stomach, helps your body break down food by releasing insulin (a hormone) into the bloodstream in amounts that match the amount of food you've consumed. Insulin is made by specialized beta-cells within the pancreas and is the key that unlocks the cell door to allow the glucose to enter. That is the only way that glucose can enter your cells, with the helping hand of insulin. In people with diabetes, the pancreas has decided to take early retirement, so less insulin is available in the body. Consequently, glucose starts to pile up in the bloodstream (hence, blood glucose), where it is then detected at abnormal levels on a blood test. These high levels of glucose in the blood eventually cause problems throughout the body because they add to the workload of the heart and other vital organs.

By the time of diagnosis, up to 80% of the

> **Some language trivia**
>
> Our word "diabetes" originally comes from the Greek word for "siphon." When blood glucose levels are high, water is pulled from the cells and put into the bloodstream, which explains why some people have increased thirst and urination as symptoms.

beta-cells may be destroyed. You can help protect your beta-cells by making healthy food choices and, when needed, using medicine. Complicating matters is the problem of insulin resistance, which is usually present in type 2 diabetes. When someone has insulin resistance, insulin is still released into the bloodstream, but the lock on the cell has changed and insulin can't open it. Obesity, lack of exercise, smoking and secondhand smoke, high blood glucose, and hereditary factors all play a role in the development of insulin resistance. Left untreated, blood glucose levels go even higher.

How did I get diabetes? I don't eat a lot of sugar.

Almost everyone would have diabetes if it just came down to how much sugar you ate. If you gain weight from consuming too many calories (whether from sugar or something else), then that can trigger diabetes if you have a genetic predisposition for it. Do you have any immediate relatives with diabetes? If you do, you have a family history of diabetes.

When asked about diabetes in the family, many people say, "No one has it in my family." But we could easily add "that you know of" to that statement. Recent studies have shown that many people have diabetes for seven years before they are diagnosed, so many people cannot be sure that their families are free of diabetes. Have any of your relatives suffered a heart attack or a stroke? Either could arise from undiagnosed diabetes. In my experience as a certified diabetes educator, the majority of people do not have any signs or symptoms of the disease. Unless you went in for a checkup *and* had a physician who knew the diagnostic criteria, your diagnosis could be missed. It happens every day. That's why it is important to know your numbers. Always ask for copies of laboratory work.

The gray zone: pre-diabetes

Pre-diabetes is a condition where the glucose levels are starting to rise but are not high enough to be categorized as type 2 diabetes. This condition often indicates that a person is at risk of developing full-blown diabetes, but he or she can lower the risk of developing diabetes by getting 30 minutes of physical activity five days a week and by losing 7% of his or her weight. Glucose values for people with pre-diabetes are:

- Fasting: 100–125 mg/dl
- Random: 140–199 mg/dl

What type of diabetes do I have?

Determining the type of diabetes you have is based on several factors: your blood glucose values, age, weight, and other laboratory tests (such as C-peptide, which indirectly shows the presence of insulin, and GAD antibodies, which show whether type 1 diabetes is developing). There are three main types of diabetes: type 1 diabetes, type 2 diabetes, and gestational diabetes.

Why did I get diabetes?

The short answer is that no one can be sure why you have diabetes. There are millions of people with diabetes, but it seems that each individual's case is different. Some scientific theories suggest that an environmental trigger activates a genetic code, flipping the diabetes switch to "on."

Is diabetes contagious?

No. You cannot catch diabetes from someone or give it to someone you know. Your relatives may have "given" it to you through your genes, but that is very different from catching a cold.

The almighty A1C

The gold standard for checking overall diabetes management is a blood test called the A1C test (also called HbA_{1c} or hemoglobin A1C). It is a blood test that measures your average blood glucose levels over a 3-month period and is represented by a percentage. The A1C test measures how much glucose is stuck to the hemoglobin part of the red blood cell. Red blood cells typically live for 2–3 months, carry oxygen and nutrients throughout the bloodstream, and carry away the waste. When a glucose molecule is nearby, it attaches to the red blood cell and won't let go; that's how we can tell what has happened for the past 3 months. Experts recommend an A1C less than 7%, which compares to an average blood glucose level of 170 mg/dl.

Type 1 Diabetes

Type 1 diabetes is an autoimmune disorder in which the body mistakenly destroys the insulin-producing islets of Langerhans, which is the cluster of beta-cells that are responsible for producing insulin. Type 1 diabetes was once called juvenile diabetes and insulin-dependent diabetes because type 1 typically affects children and young adults. But not always, which is why the name was changed.

In type 1 diabetes, the pancreas stops making insulin. Less than 100 years ago, before people with diabetes could inject insulin, a diagnosis of type 1 diabetes normally meant that death from starvation would occur in about a year. The symptoms of type 1 diabetes are typically obvious: profound thirst, urination, hunger, and rapid weight loss.

Type 2 Diabetes

A lack of insulin production *and* insulin resistance typify this disease, which used to be called adult diabetes or non-insulin-dependent diabetes to differentiate it from type 1 diabetes. Although type 2 diabetes typically arises in adults, with the biggest outbreak occurring in 35- to 45-year-olds, we now see six-year-olds getting diagnosed with type 2.

In type 2 diabetes, the body gradually makes less insulin and simultaneously becomes more insulin resistant. This means that some people with type 2 diabetes will require insulin therapy. The symptoms of type 2 diabetes are often subtle, varying from none to tiredness (especially after a large meal), blurred vision, frequent urination, and dry, itchy skin.

Gestational Diabetes

Gestational diabetes can arise during pregnancy and if left uncontrolled can cause problems with the fetus and complicate delivery. Pregnant women are typically screened for gestational diabetes at 24–28 weeks. Do you know someone who had a baby weighing more than 9 pounds? This is a condition called macrosomia and sometimes occurs in gestational diabetes. People used to think gestational diabetes went away after delivery, but now we know that it's a window into the future. Many women who develop gestational diabetes eventually develop type 2 diabetes in the next 10 years, but this can be prevented or delayed by trying to maintain a healthy body weight.

In the near future, A1C values will be reported as "A1C-derived average" or "Estimated glucose average" on your laboratory printout, so you won't have to do the math.

Because there can be different amounts of red blood cells in the body, an A1C test cannot be used to diagnose diabetes. If a person is anemic, for example, he or she will have fewer red blood cells, rendering an A1C test inaccurate. In addition, there is no national standard for the equipment used to test A1C levels.

PERSONAL GOAL

Today (date _____), I decided I can (*check one*):

☐ Acknowledge that I have diabetes.
☐ Ask my doctor's office for copies of my blood work (laboratory results).
☐ Ask to have an A1C blood test (if not done in the past 3 months).
☐ Encourage family and friends to be screened for diabetes, especially anyone over age 45.
☐ Calm my mind with three deep breaths.
☐ Other: _____.

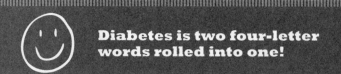

Diabetes is two four-letter words rolled into one!

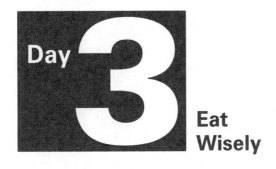

Day 3

Eat Wisely

What can I eat?

One of the keys to living successfully with diabetes is making wise food choices without compromising the joy surrounding mealtime. But it's easier said than done. We are creatures of habit. We are used to doing things a certain way. It's not about eating like a saint—it's about making small changes over time and eating wisely. Eating more nutritiously is a process, not an event. By eating healthfully, you're not following a diabetic lifestyle; you're following a healthy one.

The decisions you make about your nutrition are countless. According to a Cornell University study, people estimate that they make about 15 food and beverage decisions each day, when they actually make more than 200 such choices (e.g., decide on portion size, read the expiration date, have a cocktail, skip dessert). Much like our bodies couldn't digest a week's worth of food in one sitting, our minds need to absorb information gradually. The step-by-step guide that follows gives you small bites of information at a time. We'll start with general concepts and specific take-home points that you can start using today, with more and more details unfolding in each section. What actions are you willing to consider from the diabetes education buffet? Below are suggestions backed by research that you can incorporate into your daily life. Pick and choose the ones you want to try. Before long, you may be the healthiest eater on the block.

Eat Better and Feel the Difference!

1. After you eat, your blood glucose level goes up.
2. Foods containing carbohydrates raise glucose the most.
3. You *can* have carbohydrates, but you should stick with sensible portion sizes that are consistent.
4. Choose a variety of foods that are rich in vitamins and minerals and low in calories.
5. Eat regularly; this means three small meals a day and snacks, if needed, 2–3 hours after a meal.
6. Skipping meals can cause weight gain and fluctuations in blood glucose levels.
7. Check your glucose levels before meals and two hours after. If your blood glucose level goes up less than 50 mg/dl, your body can manage the carbohydrates in that meal.
8. Losing 5–7% of your current weight (if you are overweight) can lower glucose levels, as does a 20-minute walk.
9. Products that claim that they have "No Added Sugar" or are "Sugar Free" often still have carbohydrates! Always check food labels (the total carbohydrate amount and serving size).
10. See a registered dietitian for an individualized meal plan.

	Choose often	Choose less often
Preparation methods	Bake, broil, BBQ, steam, grill	Fried
Breads/grains*	Whole wheat, whole grains, bulgur, wild rice, brown rice, small whole-grain bagels	White bread, muffins, croissants, biscuits, white rice, French bread
Starchy vegetables*	Peas, corn, winter squash, baked/mashed/boiled potato	French fries, instant mashed potatoes
Nonstarchy vegetables	Broccoli, bell peppers, mushrooms, zucchini, celery, spinach, eggplant	Tempura or fried vegetables with added fat, vegetables in sauces
Fruits*	Whole fruits (small portions), dried fruits without added sugar	Juice: regular or with added sugar (eat fruit instead, or add water to dilute it); canned fruit with added sugar

	Choose often	Choose less often
Milk/dairy*	Nonfat plain yogurt, no-sugar-added light yogurt, nonfat or low-fat milk	Whole milk, half and half, ice cream, milk shakes, low-fat sweetened or regular yogurt
Meat and meat alternatives	Skinless, white poultry, lean beef/pork (trim off fat); fish/seafood; natural peanut butter, tofu/gluten†, legumes* (beans, peas, lentils)	Bacon, sausage, ham, luncheon meats, poultry skins, fatty meats, hard cheeses, breaded or fried fish/chicken/meats/tofu/gluten
Fats, oils, seasonings	Liquid oils (canola, olive), soft tub margarines without trans fat, nuts in small amounts, 1/8 avocado	Butter, lard, solid fats, sour cream, mayonnaise, tropical oils (palm, palm kernel, coconut)
Sweeteners, condiments*	Sugar substitutes: Splenda (sucralose), NutraSweet or Equal (aspartame), Sweet 'n' Low (saccharin); sugar-free syrups/jams/jellies	Table sugar, honey, syrup, regular jams/jellies
Desserts*, Beverages†	Water, diet sodas or other sugar-free beverages, sugar-free candies in small amounts, diet pudding, sugar-free Jell-O	Regular soda, juice, hot chocolate, donuts, pastries, cake, pie, candy, sherbet, ice cream, cookies

*Contains carbohydrates; †may contain carbohydrates.

Free Foods

Foods containing fewer than 20 calories per serving and fewer than 5 grams of carbohydrate count as a "free food" (unless you eat more than the recommended serving, in which case, they are not free). Here is a short list of free foods.

- 1/4 cup of salsa
- 1 Tbsp of salad dressing or catsup
- sugar-free gelatin or gum
- sugar substitutes
- diet soft drinks
- vinegar
- lemon juice
- seasonings
- nonfat cooking spray
- tea and coffee
- water

Getting started: A list of products

If you're lost in the grocery store, you can select from these items below. You'll still need to check serving sizes when you eat them, but they should get you off to a good start. As you continue to learn about how food choices affect your diabetes, shopping will become easier.

BEVERAGES
Calistoga waters
Crystal Light powdered drink mix
Diet sodas

DAIRY
Cheese
Alpine Lace cheese
Galaxy soy cheese
Kraft light natural cheese
Knudsen's nonfat cottage
   cheese
Laughing Cow cheese
String cheese

Ice Cream
Dreyer's or Edy's (no added
   sugar or light)
Skinny Cow frozen desserts

Milk/Yogurt
Nonfat milk and yogurt
1% low-fat milk
Soy milk
Dannon light yogurt
Promise Activ Supershot
Yoplait light

MEATS/ENTREES
Trader Joe's Just Chicken/
   Salmon
Water-packed tuna/salmon
Louis Rich cold cuts
Healthy Choice cold cuts
Butterball cold cuts

Old-fashioned peanut butter
Healthy Choice frozen meals and
   soups
Nile Spice dried soups
Morningstar frozen products
   (vegetarian breakfast links,
   patties, etc.)
Silk Tofu (soft for soup, firm for
   stir-fry)

GRAINS
Cheerios, shredded wheat,
   cornflakes
Quaker Oats cereals (hot or
   cold)
Bran cereal with psyllium
Whole-wheat bread
Whole-wheat bagels
Eggo Golden Oat waffles

SNACK FOODS
Snackwell's crackers and
   cookies
Graham crackers
Ginger snaps
Animal crackers
Vanilla wafers
Light microwave popcorn (low fat)
Rice cakes
Baked potato chips

FATS/OILS/MARGARINES
Canola or olive oil
Light mayonnaise
Light or fat-free cream cheese

Light salad dressings
Light Land-O-Lakes whipped butter
Light margarine spreads
Brummel & Brown yogurt spread

VEGGIES/FRUIT
Load up on these!

OTHER
Knott's Berry Farm no-added-sugar jelly
Smucker's low-sugar jam
Sorbet
Glucerna or Choice bars
Something trashy to read

PERSONAL GOAL

Today (date _____), I decided I can (*check one*):

☐ Make time for breakfast every day (even if it's something small).

☐ Eat every three to four hours by having three small meals a day and a little snack if I get hungry (keep that snack small; it's not a meal!).

☐ Try not to skip meals.

☐ Ask myself while eating, "Am I satisfied or stuffed?"

☐ Focus on savoring flavors.

☐ Add a serving of vegetables (fried veggies don't count!) to every meal.

☐ Limit or avoid unhealthy options such as regular soda, juice, alcohol, candy, cookies, ice cream, pastries, concentrated sweets, cakes, or anything deep fried.

☐ Select whole-wheat instead of white bread or choose fresh fruit for dessert.

☐ Replace regular sugar with a sugar substitute, such as Splenda or Equal, with recipe ideas from www.splenda.com or www.equal.com.

☐ Other: _____.

I eat often. With Barbie doll tea set dishes, I have no choice!

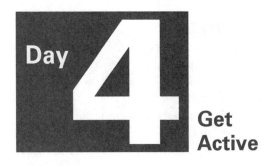

Day 4

Get Active

Who has the time to exercise? I am simply too busy.

Making time for health is challenging. You are in charge of your overall well-being. As the project manager of your health, are you making an *informed* decision when you opt out of physical activity? Exercise is the single most underutilized self-care behavior that can make a difference in all things diabetes and health in general.

Being active
- improves blood glucose levels
- improves insulin sensitivity
- helps you lose weight
- lowers blood pressure, cholesterol levels, and stress
- improves heart function, your sex life, and lets you sleep better
- keeps bones healthy
- increases lifespan (moderate activity can add two years to your life; a high level of activity can add more than four years)
- saves money (fewer health issues and less medicine mean more money in your pocket)

What kinds of activities will help my diabetes?

When it comes to adding physical activity to your lifestyle, the world is your oyster. The basic principle is to pick an activity that you enjoy, is fun, and is easy to do. The gym is great for some people; others prefer the outdoors, where they can move their bodies in the fresh air for free! Invite a friend or the entire family. If you haven't been exercising, start slowly and avoid extreme activity levels. Be sure to warm up and cool down. Going from zero exercise to an hour at the gym every day, when you haven't been to it in years, can lead to injury and discourage you from sticking with your activity plan.

PERSONAL GOAL

Today (date _____), I decided I can (*check one*):

- ☐ Take the stairs instead of the elevator.
- ☐ Get off at an earlier bus stop and walk a little farther.
- ☐ Park the car farther away.
- ☐ Stretch my muscles for five minutes in the morning.
- ☐ Walk the dog around the block.
- ☐ Do leg squats while curling my hair.
- ☐ Lift a small soup can 10 times in each hand while watching television.
- ☐ Forget about waiting for Monday to start—do it today!
- ☐ Go cherry picking.
- ☐ Other: _____.

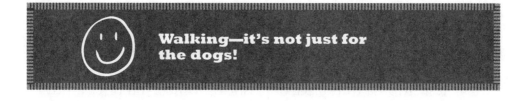

Walking—it's not just for the dogs!

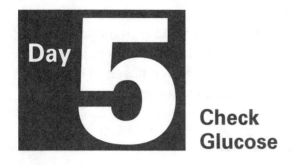

Day 5

Check Glucose

My doctor didn't say I have to poke my finger. Is it really necessary?

Self-monitoring of blood glucose (SMBG) is the best way to know on a daily basis whether you are protected against the consequences of uncontrolled diabetes. Would you get into the car without checking how much gas is in the tank? Would you withdraw money without knowing the balance of your account? Well, maybe you would if you're rich or have a chauffeur, but right now we're talking about your health. So yes, it is necessary.

What does blood glucose testing involve?

You'll need a clean pair of hands and a home blood glucose monitor kit with all of the necessary equipment, specifically:

- Blood glucose monitor—a small device that analyzes your blood glucose value within seconds.
- Lancet—a fancy name for a small needle.
- Lancet device—a fancy name for a needle holder, which helps you poke your finger or arm.
- Test strip—a thin piece of plastic on which you place a tiny drop of blood and which is placed inside the monitor.

Are you a little freaked out by the notion of needles? Good. That's normal. We'd worry if you liked needles. Luckily, the diabetes industry has vastly improved the lancing devices and everything else related to SMBG. For example, several companies advertise pain-free systems. This claim may be hard to believe, but it's true. Often, the needles are *so* small that you'll be surprised when you get a small blood sample with little to no pain. Look for small needle widths (gauge) when purchasing lancets (sizes 30 and up are narrower).

Be sure to adjust the lancet device to the necessary depth to get blood. Unless you have the strong hands of a mechanic, you won't need the deepest setting. Dial that lancet device down! Prick the side of your finger where there are fewer nerve endings and, therefore, less pain. Also, hang your hand below your heart and squeeze the base of the finger, sending more blood toward your fingertip. This makes getting a proper blood sample easier.

How do I get the right meter for me and learn how to use it?

At least 25 different meters are commercially available. How can you possibly sort through them in order to find the one that's right for you? How many features do you want on your meter? Do you need something really simple? Do you need something with an easy-to-read display? How about a meter that does not require coding? Or one that uses the smallest amount of blood? How much is cost a factor in the decision you'll be making?

Ask your health care provider for advice and a prescription for a device. Typically, you will need to speak with a health care professional who is a certified diabetes educator (CDE) and can help you sort through these questions. You can find a CDE in your area by calling 800-832-6874 or by checking the American Association of Diabetes Educators website at www.diabeteseducator.org and clicking on "Find an Educator." Or find an American Diabetes Association Recognized Education Program by visiting www.diabetes.org/education/eduprogram.asp. In addition, ask about diabetes support groups or programs at your local hospital. Don't forget that nearly all glucose meters have a 24-hour toll-free number you can call for assistance, too.

Typically, health insurance covers the equipment for home glucose monitoring, provided that you have a prescription. The best bet is to contact your health insurance provider to see whether they prefer one monitoring system (Medicare allows nearly all systems). The test strips are not cheap, and you will want to start with a system that won't hit your pocketbook too hard. Several companies provide mail-order supply delivery and bill your insurance directly. If you do not have insurance, ask your health care provider or CDE for a free monitor (which they may have depending on the meter company's sales specialists) or if they know of any other local resources.

When do I test?

You can make blood glucose testing a full-time career, but it's better not to. You can test before meals or two hours after meals, before and after exercise, before bedtime, when you change medicines, when you don't feel well, and when you feel low. Check with your health care provider about an individualized plan outlining when you should be checking. Start simple, with tests two times a day.

Option 1: Test fasting (immediately after waking in the morning) and two hours after breakfast.
Option 2: Test before dinner and two hours after dinner.

Record your results for a few weeks and look at the patterns. Are the numbers all over the place? Do you see a pattern of high glucose readings at a particular time? Ask your diabetes educator for help interpreting the numbers; otherwise, checking glucose can be an *enormous* source of frustration. Knowing what the numbers mean and how to handle them is the key to managing diabetes.

What is the target range?

In general, your blood glucose levels should fall into these ranges. However, your health care team may need to create ranges that are specific to your self-care regimen.

Before a meal: 70–130 mg/dl (called preprandial)
Two hours after a meal: less than 180 mg/dl (called postprandial)

Where can I throw away lancets?

The days of throwing lancets in the trash in solid, puncture-proof containers are numbered. You wouldn't want someone to accidentally get an injury from a lancet tossed in the trash! Instead, you'll have to check with your waste disposal company about local laws to see if a needle disposal program is available.

PERSONAL GOAL

Today (date _____), I decided I can
(*check one*):

☐ Obtain a blood glucose meter within a week.
☐ Open up that blood glucose meter kit and start
learning how to check my levels or call the toll-free
assistance line on the back of the meter.
☐ Contact a local certified diabetes educator (CDE).
☐ Test my fasting blood glucose (before breakfast) and two hours
after breakfast and record the results for a week.
☐ Test my blood glucose before dinner and two hours after din-
ner and record the results for a week.
☐ Don't beat myself up if I forget to check (as long as I don't stop!).
☐ Other: _____.

These numbers are trying to tell me something—I just wish I knew what it was!

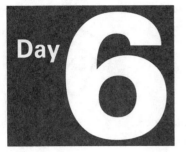

Day 6

A Tough Pill To Swallow

I don't want to start taking pills. Once you start, you never stop, right?

It's not necessarily true that you'll be taking pills forever. The key is to get your glucose levels close to or within the target ranges as quickly as possible because that will keep you as healthy as possible and help you avoid complications.

Diabetes is a progressive disease (which means that it gradually worsens over time) and typically requires some medicinal help at one point or another. If this happens, remember, you are not failing; your pancreas is. Have compassion with yourself and for your pancreas. You'd be sympathetic to a friend who has a bad heart. Apply that same kindness to yourself. If your health care team recommends medication, it's not because you have failed in your diet and exercise regimen. Instead, know that you need a little extra help to get your blood glucose to lower levels. After all, we take vitamins without much thought and buy beauty products to improve how we look on the outside. If it needs it, why not help our body on the inside, too?

PERSONAL GOAL

Today (date _____), I decided I can (*check one*):

☐ Consider that diabetes medications can help me live a longer, healthier life.

☐ Call my health care provider, CDE, or pharmacist about any medication-related questions or side effects I'm having.

☐ Take my medicines as prescribed nearly all of the time.

☐ Miss fewer doses of my medication.

☐ Develop a system to help me remember to take my medicine (for example, get a pill reminder, carry extra doses in my purse or briefcase, keep an extra dose at work).

☐ Put pills where I'll remember to take them.

☐ Write down when I take my pills to help me remember what I took.

☐ Ask the pharmacist about patient assistance programs for any of my medications (most pharmaceutical companies have financial assistance/low-cost medicine programs for qualified individuals, but you will have to jump through some paperwork hoops).

☐ Ask my health care provider if samples of my medication are available.

☐ Other: _____.

 I wanted early retirement, but my pancreas went without me.

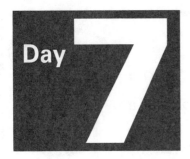

Day 7

Your Safety Net

Diabetes is overwhelming at times. How am I supposed to manage this?

Handling diabetes can be tough sometimes, especially if you try to do it yourself, but don't be afraid to ask for a little help from your friends, family, colleagues, and health care team. There is power in numbers, so remember to share the burden!

It can be a challenge finding people who are willing to be supportive to the degree that you need. You'll no doubt run into people in your immediate circle—perhaps even your partner—who don't want *anything* to do with your diabetes. To whom can you turn? Who will help you stay positive?

Decide whom to tell and whom to lean on for support. Tell them what you need. Do you want guidance about meal selections? Do you want them to go for walks with you? From a safety standpoint, you'll need to have someone who knows what to do in an emergency situation (such as what to do in case of low blood glucose, discussed next week, on p. 39). Moreover, it helps to have someone join you in your journey toward health. Who is willing to learn about carbohydrate counting with you? Who might join you in becoming more active? These are the people who may support you.

PERSONAL GOAL

Today (date _____), I decided I can (*check one*):

☐ Talk with a trusted friend or family member about my diabetes.

☐ Seek out health care professionals with whom I feel a bond.

☐ Discuss my diabetes with someone who has it to get a little more perspective. (However, be careful when you do this, because everyone has their own opinions about what a person with diabetes should or shouldn't do, some of which are medically incorrect. When getting medical advice, deal with health care professionals.)

☐ Obtain a medical alert bracelet, necklace, or wallet card as part of my safety plan.

☐ Meditate or pray for 10 minutes.

☐ Look for support in groups to which I already belong.

☐ Avoid people who will not be supportive.

☐ Be grateful for all that I do have.

☐ Other: _____.

 Sure—they help my diabetes, but what about my garage sale?

WEEK 1: REVIEW

Today's date: _____

Look back at your personal goals. How successful were you at accomplishing what you set out to do?

☐ Mostly   ☐ Sometimes   ☐ Rarely
   (80% or more)   (50–80%)   (less than 50%)

Easiest

What was the easiest to achieve? _____

_____

Why? What helped make the difference? _____

_____

How can you ensure your continued success? _____

_____

Most challenging

What was the most challenging to achieve? _____

_____

Why? What barriers got in the way? _____

_____

What can you do to remove that barrier? _____

_____

Congratulations on making it through your first week with diabetes. If you were able to make some adjustments to how you think about diabetes and your health, you are on your way. If not, the opportunity to learn is around every corner, and it is the perfect time to get started.

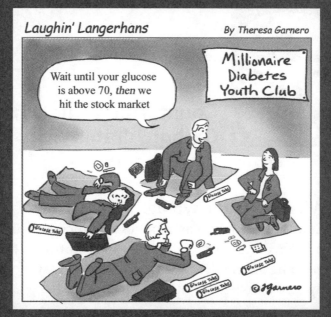

Week **2**

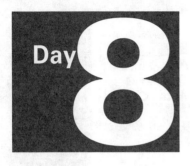

Count, Don't Cut Out, Carbohydrates

What is a carbohydrate?

Commonly known as starches and nicknamed "carbs," carbohydrates are an energy-rich nutrient found in fruits, grains, some vegetables, beans, milk, yogurt, and of course, sweets, candy, and cookies.

Why are carbohydrates important?

Carbs are the body's main source of energy. They are extra important to people with diabetes because carbs can raise blood glucose levels quickly. Once a carb enters your mouth, it converts into glucose, the fuel your entire body needs to function. Your brain needs carbs or glucose to function and think. That's why people who have glucose levels less than 70 mg/dl (called hypoglycemia—covered in day 10) can act strangely; they are running out of fuel and brainpower. All cells throughout your body depend on glucose for survival.

How can I stop eating carbohydrates? I love them!

Don't cut them out! For people with diabetes, the issue is quality and quantity. We focus on carbohydrates because they are the food group that raises glucose levels quicker than proteins. If you can control the amount of carbohydrate you eat, then you can have some control over fluctuations in blood glucose. It takes carbs only 15–90 minutes to convert into glucose in the bloodstream, whereas proteins can take hours.

The first step is to learn to identify a carbohydrate, which is the point of the exercise below. After that, you will begin learning about how carb portions affect blood glucose.

Check your carb smarts!
Circle the foods below that contain carbohydrate.

Column 1	Column 2	Column 3	Column 4	Column 5
Muffin	Grapes	Egg	Avocado	Broccoli
1/3 cup of rice	Cake	Chicken leg	Butter	Diet soda
1/3 cup pasta	Juice	Tofu	Oil	Mushrooms
1 slice whole-wheat bread	Yogurt	Cheese	Chicken skin	Salad
1 cup of milk	Corn	Fish	Nuts	Water

Answer:
Columns 1 and 2: Examples of foods and food portions with 15 grams of carbohydrate.
Column 3: Examples of protein servings only, no carbohydrate.
Column 4: Examples of fat servings, no carbohydrate.
Column 5: Examples of free foods, no carbohydrate.

How many carbohydrates can I eat?

Everyone differs slightly in how much carbohydrate they can handle. An athlete needs and can burn many more carbohydrates than someone who gets less activity. A general guideline is to have 3–4 carb choices (45–60 total grams of carbohydrate) per meal for men, 2–3 carb choices for women (30–45 total grams) per meal, and about

1 carb choice (15 grams) for snacks. A carb choice is a serving of any food that includes 15 grams of carbohydrate, and it is merely a unit of measure that helps us count carbohydrates. Your registered dietitian should let you know just how many carbohydrates you should be eating per meal.

The only way to know how many carbs are in a particular food is by looking at the food label (tips on how to read a food label are in the section below) or in a carb reference guide for foods that do not have labels (such as fruit). If counting carbs does not suit your fancy, check out the Plate Method on day 15. It's a simple way to manage carb portions without all of that counting.

Can I save up my carbohydrates from one meal to the next?

Nice try. If you missed some carbohydrates at one meal, you can't pile them up or save them for later. Eating all of those carbohydrates at one meal will have a profound impact on your glucose level. It would be too much for your pancreas to handle. Part of managing your blood glucose levels is learning how to space out your carbohydrates throughout the day.

FOOD DETECTIVE

Here's a commonly voiced concern: "I'm afraid to eat because it might hurt my body." You won't hurt your body if you know what you're putting in it. Reading the fine print will get you far when it comes to investing in your health because you'll be an informed consumer. The food label says it all, but do you know what it's saying? With a little effort, learning about the food label is one of the most powerful tools you'll use in putting together a healthy meal plan.

Just the (Nutrition) Facts, ma'am.

Food labels are like price tags. Is the food you're thinking of buying rich in nutrients or are you getting ripped off? How can you tell? Thankfully, since 1990 the federal government has required that most foods (except meat, fish, chicken, and bulk items) have a food label.

1. **Start with the serving size.** Nearly everything that is written on food packaging, including the food label, is based on the serving size. If you're not careful, you could easily double or triple your calories and fat and carbohydrate intake by eating the whole package at once. Many people mistake the package as the portion size; this is referred to as "portion distortion." Furthermore, the serving size listed on the label isn't necessarily the same serving size as you'll be using to count carbohydrates. For example, the label might say that the serving size of cooked rice is 1 cup, but a carb choice of rice is 1/3 cup.

2. **Check total carbohydrates.** Focus on the grams of total carbohydrate, not the percentage. Many people also fall into the trap of dwelling only on the sugars in a food. A product can be sugar-free and still have lots of carbohydrate (for example, sugar-free cookies made with flour). Keep it simple. Focus on total carbohydrates.

3. **Calories and calories from fat.** Here's a way to distinguish between calories and calories from fat. They are like miles per gallon in the city versus the highway. You need to know how hard your engine will work with the provided fuel. If a food choice has only 100 calories, but 85 of those calories are from fat, your arteries and waistline may suffer if you frequently choose it. The goal is to have 30% or less of total calories coming from fat. A low-calorie choice has 40 calories or fewer per serving, a moderate-calorie choice has 100 calories per serving, and a high-calorie choice has 400 calories or more per serving.

4. **Total fat, cholesterol, and sodium.** Limit these for your heart health. Try to select products with
   - less than 30% total calories from fat (divide calories per serving by calories from fat)
   - no trans fats
   - less than 300 mg of cholesterol per serving
   - less than 360 mg sodium per serving for a single item or less than 480 per entrée.

5. **Eyeball protein and check ingredients.** If your kidneys are under stress, your health care provider may suggest that you limit protein intake. So take a look at the amount of protein in the food you're evaluating and then move on to the ingredient list. Ingredients are listed in order by weight. It's likely that you won't recognize a lot of the ingredients or know what they are. Some items are vague:

- **hidden fat**—look for words like hydrogenated, oil, and shortening
- **hidden sugar**—you'll see corn syrup, dextrose, fructose, honey, juice concentrate, lactose, molasses, sucrose, and sugar alcohol
- **fat substitutes**—keep an eye out for cellulose, dextrin, emulsifier, fiber, gum, polydextrose, maltodextrin, modified food starch, olean, olestra, simplesse, and starch
- **sugar substitutes (do not contain calories or carbohydrates)**—acesulfame K, aspartame, saccharin, and sucralose

6. **Glance at % Daily Value.** This gives you an idea of the nutrient value, based on a 2,000-calorie diet. This is helpful when considering the sodium, cholesterol, and vitamin content that add up to the 100% recommended daily value.

- 20% or higher is a rich source
- 10–19% is a good source
- less than 5% is a low source

Give it a try.

Compare these Chips Ahoy cookie labels. Which one is healthier?

Chips Ahoy® baked with 100% Whole Grain:

Nutrition Facts

Serving Size 3 Cookies (33g)
Servings Per Container About 14

Amount Per Serving

Calories 150   Calories from Fat 70

	% Daily Value*
Total Fat 8g	**12%**
Saturated Fat 2.5g	**13%**
Trans Fat 0g	
Polyunsaturated Fat 2.5g	
Monounsaturated Fat 2g	
Cholesterol 0mg	**0%**
Sodium 110mg	**5%**
Total Carbohydrate 22g	**7%**
Dietary Fiber 2g	**8%**
Sugars 10g	
Protein 2g	

Vitamin A 0%	•	Vitamin C 0%
Calcium 0%	•	Iron 4%

* Percent Daily Values are based on a 2,000 calorie diet. Your daily values may be higher or lower depending on your calorie needs:

	Calories:	2,000	2,500
Total Fat	Less than	65g	80g
Sat Fat	Less than	20g	25g
Cholesterol	Less than	300mg	300mg
Sodium	Less than	2,400mg	2,400mg
Total Carbohydrate		300g	375g
Dietary Fiber		25g	30g

INGREDIENTS: WHOLE GRAIN WHEAT FLOUR, SEMISWEET CHOCOLATE CHIPS (SUGAR, CHOCOLATE, COCOA BUTTER, DEXTROSE, SOY LECITHIN - AN EMULSIFIER), SUGAR, SOYBEAN OIL, PARTIALLY HYDROGENATED COTTONSEED OIL, HIGH FRUCTOSE CORN SYRUP, LEAVENING (BAKING SODA, AMMONIUM PHOSPHATE), SALT, WHEY (FROM MILK), NATURAL AND ARTIFICIAL FLAVOR, CARAMEL COLOR.

Chips Ahoy® with real Chocolate chunks:

Nutrition Facts

Serving Size 1 Cookie (17g)
Servings Per Container About 23

Amount Per Serving

Calories 80   Calories from Fat 40

	% Daily Value*
Total Fat 4.5g	**7%**
Saturated Fat 1.5g	**8%**
Trans Fat 0g	
Polyunsaturated Fat 1.5g	
Monounsaturated Fat 1g	
Cholesterol 0mg	**0%**
Sodium 55mg	**2%**
Total Carbohydrate 11g	**4%**
Dietary Fiber Less than 1g	**2%**
Sugars 6g	
Protein Less than 1g	

Vitamin A 0%	•	Vitamin C 0%
Calcium 0%	•	Iron 2%

* Percent Daily Values are based on a 2,000 calorie diet. Your daily values may be higher or lower depending on your calorie needs:

	Calories:	2,000	2,500
Total Fat	Less than	65g	80g
Sat Fat	Less than	20g	25g
Cholesterol	Less than	300mg	300mg
Sodium	Less than	2,400mg	2,400mg
Total Carbohydrate		300g	375g
Dietary Fiber		25g	30g

INGREDIENTS: ENRICHED FLOUR (WHEAT FLOUR, NIACIN, REDUCED IRON, THIAMINE MONONITRATE (VITAMIN B1), RIBOFLAVIN (VITAMIN B2), FOLIC ACID), SEMISWEET CHOCOLATE CHUNKS (SUGAR, CHOCOLATE, DEXTROSE, COCOA BUTTER, MILKFAT, SOY LECITHIN - AN EMULSIFIER, SALT, VANILLA), SUGAR, SOYBEAN OIL, SEMISWEET CHOCOLATE CHIPS (SUGAR, CHOCOLATE, COCOA BUTTER, DEXTROSE, SOY LECITHIN - AN EMULSIFIER), PARTIALLY HYDROGENATED COTTONSEED OIL, FRUCTOSE, LEAVENING (BAKING SODA, AMMONIUM PHOSPHATE), SALT, MOLASSES, HIGH FRUCTOSE CORN SYRUP, WHEY (FROM MILK), SOY LECITHIN (EMULSIFIER), ARTIFICIAL FLAVOR, CARAMEL COLOR.

Which cookie is better? It's not so clear. The serving size is 3 of the "healthier" whole grain cookies and they have twice the calories, carbs and fat as compared to one regular Chips Ahoy. If you were able to eat just one of the regular cookies, the taste is better and you'd be better off. Unless you have the restraint of a dietitian, most people cannot eat just one cookie. You know yourself. Might be best not to have the whole box in the house!

Here's a summary comparing Yoplait yogurts.

Type	Original	Light Thick and Creamy	Whips!	Custard Style
Serving size	6 oz	6 oz	6 oz	6 oz
Total carbohydrates	33 grams	20 grams	25 grams	32 grams
Calories	170	100	140	190
Total fat (saturated fat)	1.5 grams (1)	None	2.5 grams (2)	3.5 grams (2)

Which one would you choose? The original and custard styles have the most carbohydrate, calories, and fat, so why not try the light version on your next trip to the grocery store?

Comparing food labels is a lifetime worth of discovery. This is just a simple overview to get you pointed in the right direction. Don't be intimidated by food labels. Learning how to read them is an important tool in managing diabetes. With a little time and perseverance, you'll get the hang of it.

The food label claim to fame

You'll often see eye-catching advertisements on food packages, such as "low fat" or "healthy." Do you really know what you are about to consume? These are government-approved definitions for claims made on food labels, but what do they mean? First off, remember that all of them are based on *one serving*.

Food Label Definitions

Added: at least 10% more of the Daily Value than a similar reference food

Calorie-free: less than 5 calories per serving

Cholesterol-free: less than 2 mg cholesterol per 50-gram serving of food

Extra lean: less than 10 grams of fat, 4.5 or fewer grams of saturated fat, and less than 95 mg cholesterol

Enriched: see *Added*

Fat-free: less than 0.5 gram of fat

Fewer: (whether altered or not) 25% less of a nutrient or calories than a similar reference product (e.g., pretzels can have 25% less fat than potato chips)

Fortified: see *Added*

Healthy: low in fat and saturated fat and has limited amounts of cholesterol and sodium. Single food items must also contain at least 10% of one or more of the following: vitamin A or C, iron, calcium, protein, or fiber. Sodium should be less than 360 mg per serving and less than 480 mg per serving for entrées.

Lean: less than 10% fat, 4.5 or fewer grams of saturated fat, and less than 95 mg cholesterol

Less: see *Fewer*

Low calorie: 40 or fewer calories per serving

Low cholesterol: less than 20 mg cholesterol per 50-gram serving

Low fat: 3 or fewer grams of fat

Low saturated fat: 1 gram of saturated fat or less

Low sodium: 140 mg of sodium or less

Light or lite: one-third fewer calories or half the fat of the reference food. May also describe product's texture and color.

More: see *Added*

No added salt: no salt added to the product during processing

Organic: grown or raised without synthetic fertilizers, pesticides, or hormones in a way to enhance the ecological balance of natural systems

Reduced: nutritionally altered product with at least 25% less of a nutrient or calories than the regular product

Salt-free or sodium-free: less than 5 mg of sodium

Sugar-free: less than 0.5 gram of sugar

Unsalted: see *No added salt*

Very low sodium: 35 mg of sodium or less

Zero: see *Free*

PERSONAL GOAL

Today (date _____), I decided I can (*check one*):

☐ When I am about to choose a food, ask myself, "Is that a carb, protein, or fat?"

☐ Listen to my body and how it feels after eating certain foods rather than listening to opinions about the latest diet craze.

☐ Experiment with favorite foods and dishes. Test glucose before and two hours after that meal. Record my results for further analysis in next week's section.

☐ Read at least one food label (Nutrition Facts) a day, paying attention to the portion size and carbohydrates.

☐ Put food labels on the back burner for now and instead freeze some grapes for a fun snack (10–15 grapes is the serving size).

☐ Get a carbohydrate-counting resource (check www.diabetes.org, visit www.dlife.com, or your local bookstore or library).

☐ Write down everything I eat for the next week.

☐ Measure out one cup of cooked rice to visualize what 45 grams of carbohydrate looks like.

☐ Find a local registered dietitian (RD) who can help me with an individualized plan.

☐ Other: _____.

Are you on a good label or a bad label?

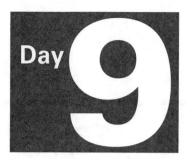

Day 9

Preparing for Activity: Shake It, But Don't Break It

Why do I need to take precautions before exercising?

Much like you'd want to have your car checked out before going on a long trip, your best bet is to get checked by your physician before you start an exercise program. You want to be sure your system can tolerate increased activity without doing any harm.

Diabetes is associated with heart disease and high blood pressure, so you and your physician should follow your blood pressure patterns. You can purchase a home blood pressure monitor to track your levels on a regular basis. For example, if your blood pressure is more than the target of 130/80 mmHg, weightlifting may not be appropriate, as it will increase your pressure and can put you at risk for a heart attack or a stroke, whereas walking would be fine. For the same reason, the eyes and kidneys are another area of concern. High blood pressure can put extra stress on the tiny blood vessels in your eyes and kidneys, which could further increase under vigorous exercise. The point is to get checked out and start with an exercise program that slowly ramps up. The last thing you need is to induce a preventable health situation or injure yourself (like pulling a muscle, twisting an ankle, etc.).

Proper foot attire is the key to preventing a host of problems. If your shoes don't fit, you'll be at risk for blisters, and if those blisters break open, you'll be at risk for infection, pain, and falls. Buy shoes that have slip-resistant soles. Your feet swell over the course of the day, so shop for them at the end of the day to make sure that shoes fit properly. Select shoes with cushioned soles and that allow room for your toes to wiggle. Wear cotton or seamless, breathable socks that don't squeeze your ankles or legs like a rubber band. Always remember to gradually break in your new footwear. Your feet will thank you at the end of the day, and you'll be more likely to enjoy longer periods of activity.

PERSONAL GOAL

Today (date _____), I decided I can (*check one*):

☐ Ask my health care provider what type and amount of exercise I can do.

☐ Slow down if I get out of breath or can't talk freely while exercising.

☐ Exercise with a friend.

☐ Wear a medical alert bracelet.

☐ Snack if my glucose is less than 100 before exercising (1/2 fruit or 1/2 sandwich) and bring glucose tablets with me if I take diabetes pills or insulin.

☐ Other: _____.

Do I get extra points for having a gardener?

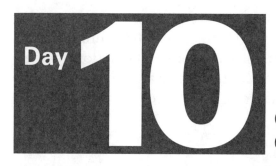

Day 10

Glucose Quantum Leaps

How low is low? What is hypoglycemia?
Hypoglycemia is the technical name for low blood glucose when readings are less than 70 mg/dl. Causes of hypoglycemia include too much medication, too little food, increased exercise without adjustments to medication, and alcohol intake. If you have more than two hypoglycemic events in one week, report it to your health care provider.

Treatment of hypoglycemia.
If you are low on sugar, you need sugar and *fast*. Follow the **Rule of 15**:

If your blood glucose is less than 70 mg/dl, take 15 grams of carbohydrate (*choose one*: 3 glucose tablets, 4 ounces of juice, 8 ounces of milk, 4 tsp of sugar, 1/4 cup of regular, non-diet soda, or a small box of raisins) and wait 15 minutes. That's the hard part. Recheck blood glucose levels. If it is still less than 70 mg/dl, take 15 more grams of carbohydrate, wait, and check again in 15 minutes. Once blood glucose rises above 70 mg/dl, have a small snack (or if it is close to mealtime, eat your meal).

Even better, follow the rule of Playing It Safe. If you are on a medication that makes your pancreas release more insulin (see day 12 for a list), carry quick-acting glucose with you at all times. It can save your life. Also, if

Symptoms of hypoglycemia

Irritability, shakiness, sweating, dizziness, rapid heart beat, profound hunger (the "mean, get-out-of-my-way" type of hunger), blurred vision, weakness, drowsiness, difficulty walking or talking. Sometimes there are few or no symptoms.

you happen to be without your monitor and suspect you are running low, when in doubt, treat for low blood glucose. If left unmonitored, it can lead to coma and death. Take the time to get some form of medical identification that will help in the event of an emergency, such as a medical alert bracelet, necklace, or wallet card.

Driving While Low

Hypoglycemia and driving can be a dangerous combination because hypoglycemia can make it hard to stay focused and can make people fall unconscious. Studies with diabetes and driving found that up to 40% of people who use insulin drive with symptoms of hypoglycemia and that 28% of people with type 1 and 6% of people with type 2 had driven with hypoglycemia in the past six months. Stay safe on the road: check your glucose levels before getting behind the wheel.

How high is high? What is hyperglycemia?

The technical name for glucose levels above 200 mg/dl is hyperglycemia. It can be caused by eating too much food, not enough medicine, stress, injury, illness, the pancreas officially retiring, or too little exercise.

Treatment of hyperglycemia

Symptoms of hyperglycemia

Feeling sleepy after eating, excessive thirst, overall tiredness, blurred vision, and frequent urination (especially in the middle of the night). Sometimes there are no symptoms.

Treating hyperglycemia is more complicated than correcting hypoglycemia. Hydration helps to dilute the high readings to a small extent, so drink some water; take extra medication, if your physician has authorized you to do so; and light exercise might help if your reading is due to consuming too many carbohydrates. Continue to test every few hours to be sure the glucose isn't headed for the moon.

Consistent readings above 250 mg/dl should be reported to your health care provider. In extreme cases, hyperglycemia can lead to coma as well.

PERSONAL GOAL

Today (date _____), I decided I can (*check one*):

☐ Keep an organized record of glucose values and a list of any comments and questions to bring to my next medical appointment.

☐ Test my glucose more often if I am under the weather, don't feel well for any reason, or have had a change in medicine.

☐ Call my health care provider when my glucose patterns do not make sense.

☐ Ask to see a diabetes specialist (an endocrinologist) to help stabilize my diabetes (check the American Association of Clinical Endocrinologists website at www.aace.com/resources/memsearch.php to find one close to your area).

☐ Make a commitment to test my glucose for as long as I have the gift of life.

☐ Give myself a mini-break from testing only when my glucose is stable and I feel great.

☐ Check my glucose at different times (such as two hours after lunch or dinner or after exercise).

☐ Test less when more than half of my glucose values are in target range for a particular time.

☐ Call my health care provider for two or more readings less than 70 mg/dl or more than 250 mg/dl.

☐ Other: _____.

After analyzing these glucose trends, I'm ready to predict the weather.

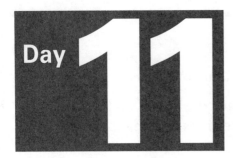

Day 11

These Feet Were Made for Walking

I don't like the look of comfortable shoes

Do you like the look of having feet? If you have lost some of the feeling in your feet because of your diabetes, then you should pay attention to what you're putting on your feet. Have you searched around for comfortable, stylish shoes? They are available, and it is a shame we have to look so hard to find them. Set foot into a shoe store and compare the number of sensible shoes versus the number of stylish shoes that will leave your feet complaining. Women's shoes are the worst. You're lucky to find a few pairs that don't bend in half or have heels guaranteed to make your chiropractor happy. Who are these designers?

What makes a good, comfortable shoe?

1. Support (you shouldn't be able to fold the shoe in two or wring it out like a towel!)
2. Cushion (you shouldn't feel the earth move under your feet)
3. Seamless across the toes (to prevent blisters)
4. Space to wiggle your toes (braiding of toes is highly discouraged)

Find a local store that specializes in diabetic footwear. You can also find a host of websites offering shoes for people with diabetes and for people who don't want to walk around in torture chambers. Stylish options are available! Check out:

- Therapeutic Footwear at www.phc-online.com (866-553-5319).
- Footwear for a healthier you with ACOR, www.acor.com (800-237-2267).
- For feet in need of special care, go to Drew Shoes, www.drewshoe.com (800-837-3739).

We take our feet for granted until something goes wrong. All it takes is a foot injury or a fall to make us notice how important our feet are. With diabetes and the loss of sensation that can arise from neuropathy (nerve damage), your feet need to be treated like royalty. Small foot problems can turn into big ones. People generally hear about the horrors of amputation and ulcers. It's one of the first things people mention when getting diagnosed, "I don't want to lose a leg." Who would? So take precautions and treat your feet right.

What about pedicures?

They sure feel great, but pedicures are not recommended for people with diabetes. Many cases of infection from pedicures have been documented. Very few pedicure establishments are ever inspected, and standards do not exist. You can ask your pedicurist about their sanitation policies and request new instruments each visit, but do you really want to risk a fungal infection that can take months to cure? Better yet, see a foot care specialist or podiatrist.

Foot care tips

- Clean your feet daily with mild soap and water.
- Dry thoroughly, especially between the toes.
- Trim nails straight across and file the corners with an emery board.
- Avoid soaking your feet (this actually dries out the skin and increases the risk of infection).
- Don't use any sharp objects on your feet (such as razor blades).
- Treat any cuts or scrapes right away with warm water and soap, apply a thin layer of antibiotic ointment, cover loosely with a bandage, and try to stay off your feet.
- Notify your doctor if any blisters do not heal within a couple of days.
- Get professional treatment for corns and calluses (don't use over-the-counter chemical corn/wart removers).
- Don't use heating pads or hot water bottles on your feet.
- Check your shoes for any debris or other unwanted objects.
- Avoid tight-fitting socks, nylons, or shoes.
- Avoid crossing your legs (this cuts off the circulation).
- Do foot exercises and stretches.
- Look for color changes, redness, tenderness, swelling, and ingrown toenails.

Safety tips while walking

Play it smart and, besides having the right kind of shoes, be aware of your surroundings. We belong to an iPod nation and are glued to our cell phones, so turn down the volume and look around at what you're walking into. Street crime, unsafe neighborhoods, and poorly maintained sidewalks can keep us inside, but if you know where you are and what you're doing, a healthy walk is not out of the question. Walk with a buddy. Plan your walking route to include safe areas. Go to the mall (but leave your credit card at home).

PERSONAL GOAL

Today (date _____), I decided I can (*check one*):

- ☐ Give up on bathroom surgery with razors, sandpaper, and pumice stones.
- ☐ Do a shoe turnaround (get rid of all those torturous shoes and replace them with comfort).
- ☐ Wear shoes. Period. Even at home, which is where most foot injuries occur.
- ☐ Check my feet every day for anything unusual (cuts, blisters, sores, calluses, broken skin, hot spots) and report anything abnormal to my health care provider.
- ☐ Remove socks and shoes whenever I see my health care provider.
- ☐ Clean my feet every day, paying attention to dry between the toes.
- ☐ Put lotion on my feet every day, except between the toes (some lotion is better than none; look for non-fragrance types with deep moisturizing qualities).
- ☐ Ask my partner for a foot rub (and give one in return)!
- ☐ Wear a stylish business suit with comfortable shoes.
- ☐ Other: _____.

 I have sweet feet!

Day 12

Sidestepping Side Effects

Many unpleasant side effects of medications can be prevented and avoided. Some medications need to be taken with meals; others on an empty stomach. Sometimes, the amount of medication prescribed can also contribute to the possibility of developing side effects. Certain medications work best by starting with a small dose and gradually building up to a certain level in your system before you notice any difference in your blood glucose levels. Others take action immediately.

Check the chart beginning on page 46 for some common oral medicines, their possible side effects, and ways to avoid them.

Type of oral diabetes medicine	Brand name (generic name)	Dosage	Timing	Possible side effects or issues
Insulin secretagogues (make the pancreas release more insulin)	**Amaryl** (glimepride)	1–2 mg a day; max 8 mg	Before the first meal	Hypoglycemia (see Day 10).
	Glucotrol (glipizide)	5 mg	30 minutes before the first meal	
		40 mg max, divided	30 minutes before breakfast and dinner	
	Glucotrol XL (extended release glipizide)	2.5–20 mg/day	Before the first meal	Hypoglycemia. Do not crush or break pill in two.
	Micronase (glyburide)	2.5 or 5 mg a day	Before the first meal	Risk for prolonged hypoglycemia in people with kidney problems or the elderly.
		max of 20 mg, divided	Before breakfast and dinner	
	Prandin (repaglinide)	0.5–2 mg	Just before meals	Do not take if you skip a meal.
	Starlix (nateglinide)	60 or 120 mg	Three times daily, before meals	
Biguanides* (limit glucose production from the liver)	**Glucophage** (metformin)	500–2,500 mg	Once or twice daily with food	Bloating, gas, and diarrhea can be minimized by taking it after a meal. Takes about two weeks to reach effective levels. Avoid use if you have kidney, liver, or heart disease or if you are elderly. Stop prior to having surgery or taking X-rays.
	Glumetza (once-a-day, extended release metformin)			

Type of oral diabetes medicine	Brand name (generic name)	Dosage	Timing	Possible side effects or issues
Thiazolidine-diones or TZDs* (reduce the body's resistance to insulin)	**Actos** (pioglitazone)	15–45 mg/day	With or without food	Can cause swelling of the ankles. Not recommended with congestive heart failure. Liver tests needed. Can take 6–8 weeks to reach full effect. Avandia may be associated with an increased risk of heart attacks and should not be prescribed for people on insulin or on nitrates.
	Avandia (rosiglitazone)	4–8 mg/day	Once or twice a day with or without food	
Alpha-glucosi-dase inhibitors (slows the absorption of carbohydrates)	**Precose** (acarbose)	25–300 mg	Taken three times a day with meals	Abdominal pain, gas, and diarrhea. If used with insulin or insulin secretagogues, hypoglycemia must be treated with pure glucose (tabs or gel) as Precose can interfere with the absorption of other carbohydrates.
	Glyset (miglitol)			
DPP-4 inhibitors (increases insulin secretion)	**Januvia** (sitagliptin)	25–100 mg	Around the same time of day, regardless of mealtime	Not to be used with sulfonylureas.
Combination medications (two types of medications in one pill)	**Avandamet** (Avandia & metformin)	Various dosing options available. Refer to specific medications listed previously.		
	Avandaryl (Avandia & Amaryl)			
	Glucovance (glyburide & metformin)			
	Janumet (sitagliptin & metformin)			
	Metaglip (metformin & glipizide)			

Known to preserve beta-cell function (in addition to exenatide, featured in month 9).

PERSONAL GOAL

Today (date _____), I decided I can (*check one*):

☐ Find out whether I take my pills before or after I eat.
☐ Tell my health care provider, CDE, or pharmacist about any possible side effects I might be having.
☐ Talk with my health care provider before stopping medications or changing doses.
☐ Keep my medicines in a temperature-controlled environment (avoid heat extremes).
☐ Check the expiration dates on my medicines.
☐ Review the written list of possible side effects of a medication provided by my pharmacist.
☐ Find out if I need to stop taking metformin before an X-ray or surgery.
☐ Report episodes of diarrhea.
☐ Report swollen feet.
☐ Other: _____.

☺ **The only side effect I feel from these medications is in my wallet.**

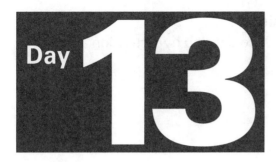

Day 13

Under Pressure

 We tend to focus on only glucose levels in people with diabetes. But do you know how many people with diabetes have high blood pressure? Nearly 70%—that's 7 in 10 people, and of those, only 5% are concerned about it! That's like only making sure your car has gas, but never changing the oil or checking the tire pressure. We need to take a step back and look at the bigger picture. What complications affect one in three people with uncontrolled diabetes? Heart attacks and strokes. That's serious business. We need to look at the three villains: high blood glucose, high blood pressure, and high cholesterol. They often travel together and are dangerous when combined.

What is blood pressure?

Blood pressure is the measurement of the force of blood as it presses against the walls of your arteries. The medical term for high blood pressure is hypertension. Hypertension puts extra strain on the heart and can damage small blood vessels in the kidneys and eyes. The blood pressure is recorded as two numbers:

- The systolic, or "top number," is the force exerted when your heart is contracting (pumping).
- The diastolic, or "bottom number," is the force present when your heart is at rest (between beats).

The target blood pressure for people with diabetes is less than 130/80 mmHg.

What causes hypertension?

In general, you are more likely to develop hypertension if you:

- have a family history
- are overweight
- don't exercise
- have unrelieved stress
- eat too much salt
- drink too much alcohol
- are African American
- smoke

You can do several things to help keep your blood pressure healthy.

- Eat wisely. Choose lots of fresh vegetables, whole-grain breads, cereals, and pasta. Avoid fried foods and those with high fat. Cut down on sodium, caffeine, and alcohol.
- Increase physical activity; do something daily.
- Manage stress.
- Stop smoking!
- Take medications (several types are available, refer to Week 7 for an in-depth list)

Have you heard about morning hypertension?

It's a condition in which average blood pressure levels taken within two hours after waking in the morning exceed 130/80 mmHg for the week. This can significantly increase your risk for stroke. One of the best ways to know your risk is to check your blood pressure at home.

PERSONAL GOAL

Today (date _____), I decided I can (*check one*):

☐ Ask my health care provider to take my blood pressure every time I go in.
☐ Keep a log of all blood pressure readings.
☐ Buy a home blood pressure monitoring device and get help in figuring out how to use it.
☐ Have a going-away party for the salt shaker.
☐ Mail my cigarettes back to the manufacturer.
☐ Ask about seeing a heart doctor (cardiologist) for my blood pressure, if I have hypertension.
☐ Find a healthy way to relieve stress.
☐ Other: _____.

You'd have high blood pressure too if you had to constantly think about diabetes.

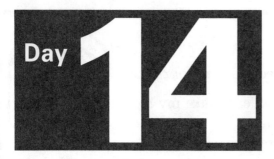

Day **14**

Stress Stop

To stress or not to stress

You've been dealing with the stress of diabetes. We know that stress can have a negative impact on life and, in particular, diabetes. What are other sources of stress in your life and how do you respond? Is there anything you can do to resolve them?

Focus on things you can change, such as food and exercise choices, how you react to others, how you spend your day, how you communicate your needs to others, how many items you put on your to-do list, and how much time you spend on any given task. Focusing on things you can't change will only add to your stress level. You can't change other people, your upbringing, the color of the stop light, your age, the number of hours in a day, a long wait for a scheduled appointment, an accident, or a death in the family.

Positive ways I can cope with my diabetes and manage overall stress

- Tell my family and friends about ways in which they can help.
- Be patient with myself.
- Shift my perspective.
- Take a different route to work or home.
- Get out and enjoy nature.
- Go for a 10-minute walk.
- Listen to the birds.
- Avoid negative people.
- Read for pleasure.
- Take things in stride.

- Celebrate life.
- Find humor every day.
- Back up computer files.
- Pick my battles.
- Keep writing in my journal.
- Do something different.
- Look forward rather than backward.
- Know my limits.
- Get enough rest and sleep regularly.
- Daydream.

PERSONAL GOAL

Today (date _____), I decided I can (*check one*):

☐ Circle one item from the preceding box to be your stress-relieving motto for the week.

☐ Other: _____.

 My diabetes is stressing me out and that's not good for my diabetes. It was easier being in denial.

WEEK 2: REVIEW

Today's date: _____

What was your track record for meeting your goals during week 2?

☐ Mostly   ☐ Sometimes   ☐ Rarely
  (80% or more)   (50–80%)   (less than 50%)

Symbol	Related Key to Diabetes Self-Management
🍎	Eat wisely
👟	Be active
📟	Check numbers (includes glucose/A1C, blood pressure, cholesterol, and weight)
🕯	Reduce stress
💊	Understand medications
↓↑	Avoid problems
👁	Reduce risks
☺	Add humor

1. Circle the one that was effortless. Focus on your triumphs.

2. Put a question mark next to the one that was troublesome. Reflect on ways you might try to tackle obstacles in the week to come.

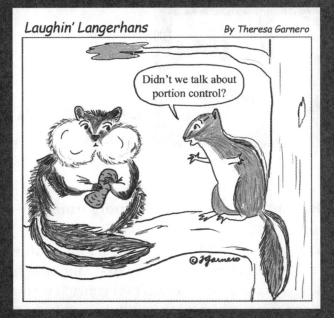

Week **3**

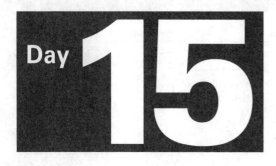

Day **15**

Let's Go Out to Eat!

How am I supposed to handle going out to eat?

With pleasure and a little preparation. Dining out is meant to be enjoyable, whether it's at a restaurant or at the house of a loved one. Take charge so you won't set yourself up for an awkward situation or unhealthy meal that will send your glucose levels through the roof.

Build a plan for success. Here are some tips for satisfying your hunger in a diabetes-friendly way:

Location, location, location. Where you go to eat makes a big difference in whether or not you'll find healthy food choices. Select the restaurant *before* you are hungry! Find ones that allow you many options or the ability to substitute menu items. Which ones offer fewer fried, lower-fat entrees? Depending on your menu selection, you might be surprised at how your glucose levels respond.

Discuss your needs. Tell your relative or waiter that you are working on making healthy food choices and ask for his or her help. You don't have to give them your full medical history to accomplish this. Whom you choose to share the diabetes news with is up to you. It may be helpful, but not essential. You can say, "I'm following smart-carb, low-fat, live-to-be-90 diet."

Be picky. Select baked, grilled, or steamed items. Avoid fried, fatty stuff. Ask for dressings and sauces on the side. Trim off fat and remove skins.

Plan for delays. Delays in getting your food can cause significant problems with hypoglycemia and/or overeating if you get too hungry. If you know dinner will be late, have a glass of milk or piece of fruit to stave off the hunger. If you are taking insulin or a medication that causes your pancreas to release more insulin, wait until the food is delivered before you take your medicine to prevent hypoglycemia.

Check portions. Serving sizes have increased by up to eight times since the 1970s, and we wonder why our waistlines are expanding! Share a meal or ask for a doggie bag right away, so when the meal arrives, you can put away half for home instead of being compelled to clean your plate. Definitely share the dessert, if you order any at all.

Experiment. Eat at your favorite haunts, and test your glucose levels before the meal and two hours after finishing to see how your body handles the meal. If your blood glucose goes up more than 50 mg/dl, try to figure out what happened by going back to the restaurant and trying a slight variation of the original order. Was it a simple case of being starved and wolfing down the entire breadbasket? Or was it a hidden honey teriyaki dressing that did it? Or how about pizza—the gift that keeps on giving? Can you identify other possible variables, such as stress (getting in an argument, being in pain, fighting a cold)? Sometimes it's not always clear, but it's worth trying to figure out why before crossing something off your list.

Leave room to breathe. Are you in touch with your belly? Do you know the point at which you go from being satisfied to being stuffed?

IS THERE AN EASIER WAY TO DO THIS?

Yes. There are two popular approaches: compare serving sizes with everyday objects and the Plate Method.

Comparing serving sizes

To get an idea of how much a recommended serving size should be for carbohydrates, protein, and fat, check the chart below and make a mental note. Does this mean that this is all you can have in a day? No. It's a visual guide of building blocks that you can use to add up your carbohydrate intake for a particular meal or snack and give you an idea about what a healthy serving size looks like.

IN THE PALM OF YOUR HAND

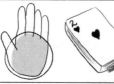 A palm or a deck of cards is about a medium-sized portion (3 ounces) of meat.

 An open hand is about 2 carbohydrate servings.

 A tennis ball is roughly the size of a medium fruit, 1 cup (45 grams of carb) of cooked pasta, 1 cup (30 grams of carb) of fresh fruit.

 A tight fist means you're good with money and also represents about 1 carbohydrate serving of cooked cereal or ice cream.

 The tip of your thumb is about 1 serving of fat (such as oil or mayonnaise).

 A large egg represents 1/4 cup of raisins.

   A size C battery or 4 dice is the serving recommendation for low-fat or fat-free cheese.

The Plate Method

Originally described in the Swedish magazine *Van Naring* ("Our Nourishment") in 1970 and transformed into a patient booklet by Swedish nutritionists in the early 1980s, the Plate Method was adapted by the Idaho Diabetes Care and Education practice group in 1993. Since then, it has helped many individuals with diabetes navigate the issue of deciding what to eat. Below is a simplistic adaptation to help you get started.

The Plate Method requires basic knowledge about food groups. Not all plates are created equal; that's why it's vital to use a nine-inch plate with this method. Let's divvy this up to give you a visual. Please refer to the special instructions that follow the chart.

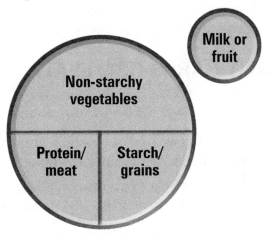

FOOD GROUPS AND SERVING SIZES

Nonstarchy Vegetables: Fill half of your plate with one to two servings of nonstarchy vegetables (if you want to have potatoes, peas, corn, or winter squash, count them as a starch, not vegetables). Examples: 1/2 cup of cooked or 1 cup raw broccoli, spinach, carrots, beets, green beans, cauliflower, zucchini, bell peppers, mushrooms, lettuce, celery, tomato, or cucumber.

Protein/Meat: One serving is about 3–4 ounces of fish, lean meat, or chicken and should take up a small portion of the plate (about 1/4). Beans, lentils, or tofu count as 1 carb and lean meat choice. Examples: 1 ounce of white turkey or chicken, tuna (packed in water), halibut, shrimp, scallops, salmon, fat-free cheese, pork, beef, egg (limit yourself to three per week), or veggie patties.

Starches/grains: Fill up about 1/4 of the plate. Examples: a small potato, 1/3 cup pasta, small bowl of soup or cereal, 1 slice of bread, 1/2 English muffin, 1/2 cup of beans, peas, or corn. You can double the starch/grain serving sizes if you trade the milk or fruit choice for a snack later.

Milk: Use a small cup (4 ounces); low-fat and nonfat milk are best.

Fruit: Choose one small piece of fruit or a small bowl of berries or melon. Examples: apple, small banana, kiwi, orange, peach; 1 cup raspberries/strawberries, 3/4 cup blueberries, or 15 grapes.

Snacks: Snacks may or may not be needed based on your hunger level, blood glucose levels, and weight loss plans. Have a snack before bedtime if your blood glucose is less than 120 mg/dl.

HOW MANY CARBS CAN I EAT?

Depending on your after-meal blood glucose values and weight-management goals, use this as a beginning guide:

Women: Start with two or three carb choices* per meal.

Men: Start with three or four carb choices* per meal.

*1 carb choice = 15 grams of carbohydrate (e.g., 1 slice of bread, 1 cup of milk, 1/3 cup of pasta or rice)

Of course, the best option is to meet with a registered dietitian first. He or she can tell you exactly how many carbs you can eat.

WHAT ABOUT ALCOHOL?

Adding alcohol to diabetes is a big gamble. Diabetes is unpredictable by itself, and alcohol can make blood glucose levels change unpredictably. If you don't drink alcohol, now is not the time to start. However, if you can afford the extra, empty calories and risk of weight gain that drinking alcohol brings, consider using the following tactics to turn a gamble into a calculated risk.

- Play it safe, and get your doctor's blessing.
- Check your blood glucose before drinking.
- Have some sort of food with the alcohol (whether it's a meal or some hors d'oeuvres).
- Sip your drinks slowly and consider alternating with water and/or non-alcoholic drinks.
- Know what constitutes *one* drink (12 ounces of beer, 5 ounces of wine, 1 1/2 ounces of liquor).
- Know *your* limit (moderate consumption for women is no more than 1 drink a day; for men, no more than 2 per day, but

this does not apply to *all* women or *all* men).

- Alcohol consumed in the evening may cause hypoglycemia after breakfast the next day (especially when combined with after-breakfast exercise).
- Alcohol can reduce your judgment and ability to recognize and react to hypoglycemia.
- Bring supplies for treating hypoglycemia, just to be prepared.
- Limit or avoid sweet alcoholic beverages with fruit juice/high-sugar content.
- Count one alcoholic drink as 2 fat servings.
- Avoid drinking when your diabetes is not well controlled.

HEALTHY CHOICES WITH ETHNIC FOODS

Do the menus at ethnic restaurants sometimes make it hard to choose the healthiest options? Here are some tips for making healthy choices.

Type	Healthier Options	Try to Avoid
Chinese	Vegetable dishes; order items for the whole table and share; sauces on the side; low-sodium soy sauce; use chopsticks!	Fried rice; noodles; egg rolls; items described as "crispy," "golden brown," or "sweet and sour"; regular soy sauce
Indian	Chicken tikka masala, shrimp bhuna, fish vindaloo or tandoori-prepared chicken, baked pappadam bread	Fried appetizers; coconut oil; naan; chapatti; roti; ghee (clarified butter); malai (a thick cream)
Italian	Antipasto dish with baked veggies; insalata caprese; share a pasta and salad dish; pasta dishes with a tomato sauce (puttanesca, arrabbiata, vongole); grilled or "griglia"	Garlic bread; bread and butter; pizza (limit yourself to 2 slices and add salad); Alfredo or primavera sauces; items listed as "carbonara," "frito," "saltimbocca," "parmigiana"
Mexican	Pinto or black beans; fajitas (you decide what goes in them); side salad instead of rice	Fried tortilla chips; beef or cheese burritos; sour cream; fried taco shells; Spanish rice
Thai	Broth-based soups; stir-fried, grilled, or steamed dishes; baked or steamed tofu and vegetables	Thai iced tea; dishes made with coconut milk; fried dishes

PERSONAL GOAL

Today (date _____), I decided I can (*check one*):

☐ Practice stopping eating a few bites earlier
than I normally would.

☐ Go for a walk to gather menu information on
local restaurants (to get ideas of where and what to eat) or
check out the National Restaurant Association's website at
www.restaurant.org/dineout/nutrition.cfm.

☐ Order salad dressing, sour cream, butter, and gravy on the side.

☐ Turn down the "Do you want cheese with that?" offer.

☐ Avoid foods prepared with the words "breaded," "crispy," or
"creamy."

☐ Request food that is baked or broiled rather than fried.

☐ Ask for a to-go container for half of my order before it arrives.

☐ Graciously pass on offers of unhealthy food.

☐ Other: _____.

☺ **I only had _one_ glass of wine;
I just kept filling it up!**

Day 16

Every Step You Take

 You don't have to enroll in an extreme sport to reap the benefits of physical activity. It's the everyday steps you take that can make a world of difference. Did you know that lack of exercise is a major risk factor for heart disease and stroke? More than 60% of adults in the U.S. do not get enough activity and at least 25% are completely inactive during their leisure time. Not getting regular activity is like parking the car in the garage for years and then being surprised when it doesn't start or function normally. We need to run our engines regularly to maintain maximum performance.

Challenge yourself to get more steps every day. Invest in a pedometer (a small battery-powered device that clips to your waistband and counts steps). A pedometer is just the ticket to raise your awareness of how many steps you're actually taking and provides motivation to get more activity in your daily plan. Try to get to 10,000 steps a day.

The Benefits of Walking

- Adding 2,000 steps a day can prevent weight gain and can prevent diabetes.
- Taking 2,000 steps burns about 100 calories.
- Americans as a whole average about 5,600 steps a day and have an obesity rate of 22.8%.
- People in Colorado average about 6,500 steps a day, the highest rate in the U.S., and have an obesity rate of 16%.
- The Amish average about 16,000 steps a day and have an obesity rate of 9%.

Where can I get a pedometer?

You can find pedometers at your local pharmacy or on the Internet. Omron (www.omronhealthcare.com) makes an accurate, easy-to-use pedometer that keeps daily averages for a quick comparison of walking trends. The Yamax Digi-Walker pedometers (www.new-lifestyles.com) are also very good. Regardless of the brand you select, make sure it has—and that you use—a security strap feature to prevent the pedometer from falling off your clothes. Losing pedometers can become an expensive habit to support.

Do I need to get my walking in all at once?

The U.S. Surgeon General recommends 30 minutes of moderate daily activity, and it doesn't have to be all at once. The same benefit is achieved in three 10-minute increments. If you want to lose weight, aim for 60 minutes a day.

Is running better than walking?

Not necessarily. Walking briskly can provide the same health benefits as running. Runners tend to have more injuries and can miss more days of activity.

Is it okay to use hand weights while walking?

No way! Leave the hand weights at home. Hand weights can increase blood pressure, which can be dangerous. You should do your weight training separate from walking.

PERSONAL GOAL

Today (date _____), I decided I can (*check one*):

☐ Buy a pedometer and measure the number of steps I take every day.

☐ Stretch before I walk.

☐ Start a program of 10 minutes of brisk walking three days a week.

☐ Gradually increase the amount of steps I take on a weekly basis.

☐ Increase to 30 minutes of walking per day at least five days a week.

☐ Walk while running errands rather than relying on my car.

☐ Check out www.americaonthemove.org to find activities in my community.

☐ Write my daily steps on a calendar, so I can watch my progress.

☐ Don't quit if I miss a few days.

Walk a mile in his shoes? No thanks. I'd rather walk two in mine.

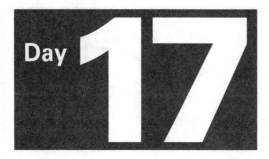

Day

Sweet Memories

What does that "M" button on my glucose meter do?

"M" is for memory, "T" is for Technology, and "H" is for Help! Blood glucose monitors offer advanced functions that make it easier to identify trends. The memory function is standard with most systems, and data management software programs are usually available for most monitors. These programs are an excellent way to help keep track of your numbers and to display your results in easy-to-read charts.

Some glucose monitor companies allow you to download their software for free; instead, they usually charge you for the cable that makes it possible to use the software. How do you know if your system has this option? Flip your meter over, get out a magnifying glass to read the number for the toll-free assistance line on the back, and call to ask. You can also check your monitor company's website. If you can use these programs, they are extremely helpful in managing your diabetes.

What if I don't want to use a computer?

If that's the case, use the logbook that came with your meter or ask the meter company to mail you another paper logbook. Many people also create their own personal systems, like using a columned accountant's notebook. It doesn't really matter, as long as the information is organized and you and your health care provider are able to interpret the data. Consistently writing down your results is the best way to see potential areas of concern that you might not notice otherwise. By looking at patterns, you can learn to anticipate and solve problems ahead of time.

Does my meter tell me my A1C?

Although there are meters that exclusively check A1C levels, most glucose monitors do not determine A1C. You can use the memory averages on a regular glucose monitor to get a general idea about your A1C, but it's nowhere near as accurate as an A1C test. Many glucose monitors automatically calculate glucose averages with the push of a button (typically 14- or 30-day averages), but that average is only as valid as the numbers available. So, if you only test in the morning, when glucose values tend to be on their best behavior, you will get an average that is fantastic but probably not realistic. The chart below shows how average glucose levels correlate to A1C levels.

A1C (%)	Average glucose	A1C (%)	Average glucose
6	135	10	275
7	170	11	310
8	205	12	345
9	240		

What was your last A1C test result?_____ Date: _____

PERSONAL GOAL

Today (date _____), I decided I can (*check one*):

☐ Check out my meter's memory functions.
☐ Ask my local pharmacist or CDE about the functions on my meter.
☐ Check my blood glucose before and two hours after breakfast or another meal.
☐ Contact my meter's manufacturer and ask for more information about connecting it to a computer.
☐ Ask someone to help me set up my software program.
☐ Print out a copy of my recent blood glucose values.
☐ Keep a consistent, organized record of my blood glucose values.
☐ Other: _____.

Thanks to A1C goals, I can strive to be below average.

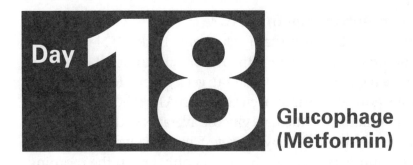

Day 18

Glucophage (Metformin)

Who takes this drug?
People with type 2 diabetes.

What is Glucophage?
Glucophage is the brand name for metformin, which is the generic name. Metformin has been used in Europe since the 1960s and became available in the U.S. a few decades later. It belongs to the biguanide class of medications and is available in pill and liquid forms and in combination pills. It can be taken in combination with other diabetes medications, including insulin.

How does this drug work?
Metformin works by decreasing the amount of glucose production from the liver. It does not cause weight gain and can help lower triglyceride levels. It may also preserve beta-cells. It is taken with or toward the end of a meal. Visible changes in blood glucose levels may not be seen until after two weeks of consistently taking the drug.

Possible side effects
Bloating, gas, nausea, and diarrhea (usually subsides after the first week).

Warning
If you have a liver problem (such as hepatitis), drink excessive amounts of alcohol, have kidney disease, or have a history of heart failure, metformin is *not* for you. It should be used cautiously with people over 80 years old. Your doctor will probably request lab tests to check kidney and liver function before starting you on metform-

in. A rare, but often fatal, condition called lactic acidosis can occur in certain high-risk groups.

PERSONAL GOAL

Today (date _____), I decided I can (*check one*):

☐ Limit alcohol when on metformin (check with my doctor to see if it's okay to have an occasional drink, but stay hydrated when enjoying a little alcohol).

☐ Take my medication as prescribed.

☐ If I miss a dose of metformin, I'll take it if I am still within three hours of the scheduled dose (with a snack). If more than three hours have passed since my scheduled dose, I'll skip that dose and take my prescribed dosage at the next scheduled dose. However, I won't double up on doses (i.e., take two pills at the next scheduled dose) if I miss one.

☐ Continue to take metformin if my glucose is in target range, unless my doctor advises otherwise.

☐ Tell my health care provider if I stop taking my medication, regardless of the reason.

☐ Call my provider to report diarrhea, gas, nausea, or bloating that does not go away.

☐ Other: _____ .

I love what you do for me, metformin!

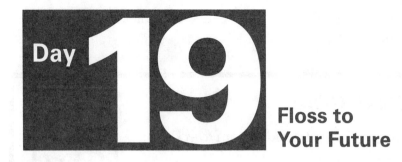

Day **19**

**Floss to
Your Future**

**Isn't dental care important for everyone?
What's different for people with diabetes?**

People with diabetes have a higher rate of gum disease and teeth problems than the general public. There is a direct link between gum disease and increased mortality rates from cardiovascular and kidney disease. Keep your teeth and gums clean and you will help keep your heart and kidneys happy.

Controlling blood glucose levels is the best way to prevent tooth and gum problems. Brushing and flossing your teeth helps protect them against plaque and other problems. When your blood glucose levels are consistently high, your gums become an ideal location for bacteria to collect. If this leads to an infection, your blood glucose levels may go even higher, reducing your ability to heal. If bacteria hang out in the gum margin, you may develop gingivitis, a condition that causes the gums to be inflamed and bleed. Left to fester, this can lead to periodontal disease, a chronic inflammatory disease that destroys the gums and bones and can lead to tooth loss. This doesn't happen overnight, so start taking care of those choppers.

Signs and Symptoms of Periodontal Disease

- Red, swollen, tender, or bleeding gums.
- Gums that have receded from the teeth.
- Ongoing bad breath.
- Loose teeth.
- Pus comes out when the gums are pressed.
- Changes in how the teeth fit together.
- Usually not painful for the person with diabetes.

Dry mouth

Dry mouth can cause tissues in your mouth to become swollen and sore, and it may occur due to hyperglycemia, dehydration, neuropathy, and medication side effects. Drinking water, sucking on sugar-free candies, or chewing sugar-free gum may help. Your dentist may suggest an artificial saliva substitute as well. Dry mouth can lead to thrush, a fungal infection technically termed candidiasis, which appears as sore white or red areas throughout the mouth and tongue. Prescription medications are available for thrush.

What if I have dentures?

Even with full dentures, it is important to brush your gums, your tongue, and the roof of your mouth every morning before putting in your dentures. To help keep your gums clean, rinse out your mouth with lukewarm saltwater. Check with your dentist about the proper brush and cleaning solution for your dentures. Remember not to use regular toothpaste because it can scratch dentures.

PERSONAL GOAL

Today (date _____), I decided I can (*check one*):

- ☐ Call the dentist for a checkup.
- ☐ Tell my dentist I have diabetes.
- ☐ Use only toothpaste with fluoride.
- ☐ Get a new, soft-bristle toothbrush.
- ☐ Consider purchasing an electric toothbrush.
- ☐ Brush my teeth for at least two minutes and at least twice a day.
- ☐ Floss my teeth daily.
- ☐ Tell my dentist about ill-fitting dentures, if I have them.
- ☐ Brush my tongue after I brush my teeth.
- ☐ Other: _____.

Smile and the world wonders what you're up to.

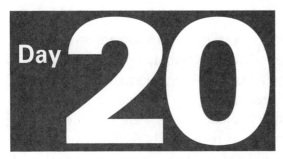

Day **20** Illness

Why did my glucose go up when I had the flu? I didn't eat anything.

We tend to think that what we eat is the only way our blood glucose levels rise. However, under periods of stress, our fight-or-flight hormones (such as adrenaline) give our bodies extra energy to defend ourselves (or run away). Extra glucose pours in from the liver to give the body extra energy to fight off attackers, regardless of whether that attacker is a bear or a bacteria or a virus. Pain also causes a release of stress hormones, as does emotional stress.

Your glucose can be stabilized for years until you catch a cold. It is in your best interest to be hypervigilant about your diabetes management when you are ill. Staying on top of your glucose values by testing more often than you usually do (at least every four hours) can mean the difference between a visit to the physician's office and a trip to the hospital.

What if I am too sick to eat?

Your body still needs energy during periods of illness. You may not be able to follow your meal plan if you are feeling nauseated.

Seriously, Get a Flu Shot

Make sure you get a flu shot every year. Fifty percent of people with diabetes do not get one, even though they are three times more likely to die from the flu. Vaccinations typically begin in October. Ask your health care provider where you can get a flu shot. It can save your life.

In situations like this, try eating foods high in carbohydrate. That way, you'll still get some energy from your meals, even if they're tiny. Examples of foods to choose when you are sick include:

- 1 cup of soup or noodles
- 1/2 cup of regular soda
- 1/2 cup of juice
- 6 saltine crackers
- 1/2 cup of ice cream

Try to stay hydrated because dehydration can make your blood glucose levels go crazy. Drink calorie-free liquids, such as water, tea, and broth.

At what point should I be worried and call the doctor?

Contact your health care provider if you have a persistent fever, nausea or vomiting, diarrhea that lasts more than six hours, blood glucose levels less than 70 mg/dl on any given day that you are sick, or blood glucose levels more than 250 mg/dl for two consecutive days. Ask your health care provider when he or she should be called.

Have a sick-day plan.

The best way to avoid problems when you're sick is to have a plan. Stock up with some key items, so you will be prepared for most situations. Have sugar-free cough drops and fever medicine available. Have a list of contact information for your health care providers handy so you can call if you have questions. You'll also need to have a plan for handling your medications when ill. You may need to change your dosages. Discuss these issues with your health care team beforehand, and you will avoid many unexpected surprises.

PERSONAL GOAL

Today (date _____), I decided I can (*check one*):

☐ Stock up on supplies that I might need when I am ill, such as sugar-free cough drops, fever medicine, over-the-counter pain medicine (that has been approved by my physician), soup, saltine crackers, small boxes of juice, tea, and other beverages.

☐ Check my blood glucose at least every four hours when I don't feel well.

☐ Call my health care provider when my blood glucose levels are above 250 mg/dl for more than two days or if I have one reading of less than 70 mg/dl.

☐ Ask my health care provider about how to handle medications during periods of illness.

☐ Put together a list of important phone numbers, so I am prepared if I need to make an emergency call.

☐ Take a sick day from work if I am ill.

☐ Conserve my energy.

☐ Drink plenty of calorie-free fluids.

☐ Other: _____ .

Why do I have to be sick to enjoy a little guilt-free ice cream?

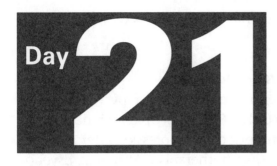

Day 21

From Depression To Refreshin'

 How's your mood? What do you do for fun? Have you always loved going to the movies or getting out in nature? If you've suddenly found that you couldn't care less about the things that you used to love, that's a sign of depression. Depression is serious business in people with diabetes. People with diabetes who are depressed can avoid or neglect their self-care management (such as not taking medications or not checking blood glucose levels regularly) and endanger themselves.

What is depression?

Depression is much more than occasionally feeling blue or being sad. According to experts Dr. Lustman and Dr. Clouse, depression is a syndrome with nine symptoms, at least five of which need to be present nearly every day for at least two weeks. Take a look at the list below and see if any of these apply to you on a regular basis.

One of these:
- Depressed mood
- Loss of interest and pleasure

Plus four of these:
- Change in sleep patterns
- Change in appetite or weight
- Low energy or fatigue
- The body doesn't want to do what the mind tells it to do
- Lack of concentration
- Thoughts of suicide or death

Does any of this sound familiar? If so, seek help from your health care team. People with diabetes have a higher risk of becoming depressed.

I don't need to see a psychotherapist.

People often groan at the mention of psychotherapy, but consider this: a scientific study showed that 85% of people with depression and diabetes reported no more episodes of depression after 10 weeks of hour-long sessions with a psychotherapist. Although psychotherapy is often socially stigmatized, it is simply best way to deal with depression.

Benefits of treating depression

- No more depression
- Improved sleep and eating patterns
- Reduced pain
- Increased social and physical activity
- Better coping ability
- Improved blood glucose control

PERSONAL GOAL

Today (date _____), I decided I can (*check one*):

☐ Go out and be with people today.
☐ Do for myself what I would normally do for someone else.
☐ Get out for at least a five-minute walk or a breath of fresh air.
☐ Forgive myself for any mistakes I've made.
☐ Strive for consistency, not perfection, with my diabetes self-care.
☐ Find a therapist (ask my health care team and insurance company, contact the Mental Health Association at 800-969-6642 or www.nmha.org/affiliates/directory/index.cfm, or talk with my school counselor, minister, rabbi, or imam).
☐ Check my insurance coverage for mental health care.
☐ Call the National Hopeline Network Crisis Center at 800-784-2433 if I need help immediately.
☐ Discuss symptoms of depression with my health care providers.
☐ Other: _____.

I'm so bummed I couldn't care less, but I end up caring about being so bummed.

WEEK 3: REVIEW

Today's date: _____

You made it to the magical three-week point. By now, some of the changes you've brought into your life to help manage your diabetes will have become good habits.

Flip back through the past 3 weeks of your personal goals and review.

1. Which goal was completed without much thought or effort?

_____

_____

2. Which goal did you forget that you had made? _____

_____

3. In which area did you surprise yourself with your ability to manage? _____

_____

4. What self-care behavior was a struggle and why? _____

_____

_____

5. What would you like to focus on for the next week? _____

_____

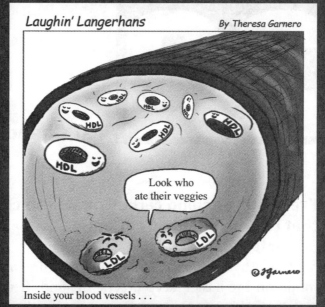

Week 4

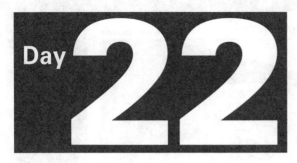

Day 22

Fat Chance

I've been watching carbohydrates so closely that I haven't paid any attention to cholesterol.

Learning about healthy nutrition is like understanding a new language. You build on the basics, keep practicing, and then one day you find yourself speaking in that new language. You become confident and knowledgeable and keep learning new words or phrases. Diabetes self-management, and in particular nutrition, is similar. We become wiser or risk getting wider. If you try to assimilate all of the components of sound nutrition at the same time, it *is* overwhelming. That's when people throw in the towel and say, "Forget it."

What is cholesterol?

Cholesterol is a waxy substance made by the liver that moves through your bloodstream and helps your cells function. Your body usually makes all of the cholesterol it needs, but your food choices add extra cholesterol to the bloodstream and contribute to extra fat buildup within the arteries. Adding high cholesterol to uncontrolled diabetes and high blood pressure can turn things into a ticking bomb, so let's turn our focus to decreasing fat consumption and stop that ticking clock!

Fats, fats, and more fats!

Remember that *all* fats carry *twice* the number of calories as carbohydrates or protein. Try to limit your total fat intake so that it constitutes less than 35% of the total calories you take in every day. But you should also know your fats, because there are several different kinds. Here are some of the healthier fats and ones to limit or avoid.

Healthier Fats (can lower blood cholesterol)

Monounsaturated fats are found in olive, canola, and peanut oil; avocados; seeds; and most nuts, such as almonds, peanuts, cashews, and hazelnuts.

Polyunsaturated fats are found in sunflower, safflower, corn, soybean, sesame, flaxseed, and cottonseed oils; some fish (such as salmon, mackerel, albacore tuna, sardines, and trout); and walnuts.

Avoidable Fats (can raise blood cholesterol)

Saturated fats are found in animal products (including dairy, chicken, eggs, meat) and tropical oils (coconut, cocoa butter, and palm). They are usually solid at room temperature.

Trans fats or hydrogenated fats are found in most baked goods, cookies, pastries, pies, fast foods, shortening, and stick margarine. They also lurk in most processed foods (look for "hydrogenated fats" on the label). Trans fats are sometimes called trans fatty acids.

What are omega-3 and omega-6 fats?

The omega fats are called essential fatty acids because you can only get them from your diet. Most omega-3 fats are found in fish. Other excellent sources are walnuts, flax seeds, and pumpkin seeds.

Omega-6 fatty acids help to either block or promote inflammation in major body systems (like the cardiovascular, circulatory, neurological, and gastrointestinal systems). Good sources of omega-6 are whole-grain breads, poultry, eggs, cereal, and some vegetable and seed oils. Unfortunately, all that yummy junk we love so much is also loaded with not-so-friendly omega-6 fats: cookies, candy, cake, fast food, fried food, crackers, and chips.

Consuming more omega-6 than omega-3 puts the body more at risk for conditions like heart disease, cancer, high blood pressure, diabetes, and arthritis. Studies show that to stay healthy, our diets should have an even balance of omega-3 and omega-6 fats. What does this mean? Eat more fresh foods and veggies like broccoli, cauliflower, kale, cabbage, and Brussels sprouts. Plus, it never hurts to choose nonfat milk.

Smart choices for healthy cholesterol

CHOOSE OFTEN*			
Helps improve your cholesterol levels			
Olives	Peanut oil	Broccoli	Salmon
Olive oil	Avocados	Zucchini	Mackerel
DAG oil†	Nuts (almonds, peanuts)	Chard	Sardines
Canola oil	Spinach	Oils (sunflower, soybean, cottonseed)	Tuna

*In a low-fat diet. Too much of any fat can increase your cholesterol.

†DAG oil is composed predominantly of diacylglycerols (or diglycerides) from soybean and canola oils (under the brand name Enova). This oil may offer health benefits not offered in other oils (less of it is stored as fat compared to vegetable oil, and it may therefore help reduce weight and A1C levels).

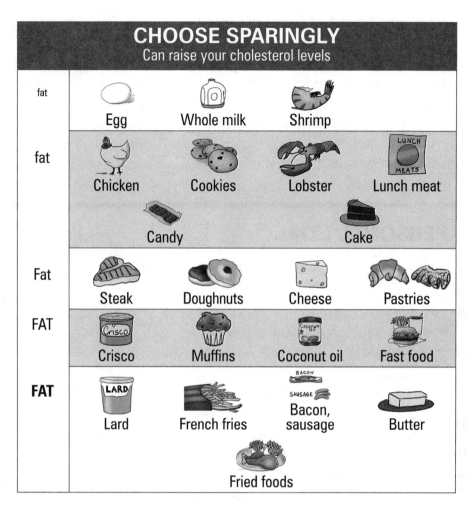

CHOOSE SPARINGLY
Can raise your cholesterol levels

fat	Egg	Whole milk	Shrimp
fat	Chicken	Cookies	Lobster	Lunch meat
	Candy		Cake
Fat	Steak	Doughnuts	Cheese	Pastries
FAT	Crisco	Muffins	Coconut oil	Fast food
FAT	Lard	French fries	Bacon, sausage	Butter
		Fried foods		

What's better: butter or margarine?

Check out this chart and decide which.

Comparison of Butter and Margarines (1 Tbsp)

	Butter	Stick margarine	Tub margarine	Smart Balance	Benecol
Calories	110	100	60	80	70
Fat	12 grams	11 grams	7 grams	9 grams	8 grams
Saturated Fat	8 grams	2.5 grams	1.5 grams	2.5 grams	1 gram
Trans Fat	0	3 grams	0	0	0
Cholesterol	30 mg	0	0	0	0

Source: The Diabetes Carbohydrate & Fat Gram Guide, *by Lea Ann Holzmeister, RD, CDE.*

Have you heard of plant sterols?

Plant sterols are components of cell membranes in many fruits, legumes, nuts, seeds, and vegetables. Many recent studies have shown that plant sterols can lower your cholesterol levels. It can be a challenge to add plant sterols to your diet, but you can find many foods, beverages, and dietary pills that contain plant sterols. This may be a good addition to a healthy eating plan, but be sure to check with your registered dietitian first.

PERSONAL GOAL

Today (date _____), I decided I can (*check one*):

☐ Switch to a lower-fat (1% or 2%) or fat-free milk.
☐ Eat less cheese or switch to low-fat cheese.
☐ Avoid bacon, sausage, and other fatty meats.
☐ Remove the skin from poultry.
☐ Double the amount of fresh vegetables in my diet.
☐ Ask for the salad dressing on the side.
☐ Keep both olive and canola oils in the kitchen (canola has omega-3 fat and both are monounsaturated fats).
☐ Cut down on pastries, cakes, cookies, and junk food.
☐ Limit eggs yolks to two per week (the egg whites are the healthy part).
☐ Other: _____.

 These pants no longer fit my trans fanny.

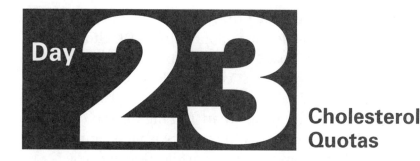

Day **23**

Cholesterol Quotas

My doctor watches my cholesterol. My numbers must be OK.

Are you sure? That's like handing your taxes over to an accountant and not finding out if you will pay extra or get a refund. Don't you want to know if you are at risk for heart disease?

Elevated levels of cholesterol and high blood pressure are a double threat to your heart. Knowing your numbers is the first step toward maintaining your health. Typically, high cholesterol has no symptoms, so your best bet is to have a lipid panel (a simple blood test) taken to evaluate your cholesterol status.

Okay, so what's total cholesterol?

Don't waste your efforts concentrating on total cholesterol. It doesn't give you the detail you need. Think of total cholesterol like a class you took in school that only graded with a Pass or Fail. You can say you passed a course without knowing that you just squeaked by with a C-minus. In general, you want your total cholesterol to be less than 200 mg/dl.

HDL cholesterol stands for Healthy.

The HDL stands for "high-density lipoprotein." HDL cholesterol is known as the "healthy" or "good" cholesterol because it lowers the levels of "bad" or "lousy" cholesterol. Ideal levels are more than 40 mg/dl for men and more than 50 mg/dl for women. You can raise your HDL cholesterol level by being active on a regular basis, controlling your weight, and quitting smoking.

LDL cholesterol stands for Lousy.

The LDL stands for "low-density lipoprotein." LDL cholesterol is known as the "lousy" or "bad" cholesterol because is clogs up the walls of your arteries with small, sticky particles of cholesterol. This is often called plaque and can lead to strokes and heart attacks. Ideal levels for LDL cholesterol are less than 100 mg/dl. You can lower your LDL cholesterol levels by eating foods with less saturated fat, trans fat, and cholesterol and by taking medication, if needed.

What are triglycerides?

Triglycerides are considered free fatty acids, which can be very useful in the body at appropriate levels, but are harmful if levels rise above 150 mg/dl. You may see "triglycerides" shortened to TG on lab reports. The current recommended level for triglycerides is less than 150 mg/dl. You can lower your triglyceride level by drinking less alcohol, eating less sugar and white starches or grains, and keeping your blood glucose under control. Medication may be needed.

How often do I need to have my cholesterol checked?

For adults, check fasting lipid levels at least once a year. Some health care providers will want to monitor lipid levels four times a year until goals are reached.

PERSONAL GOAL

Today (date _____), I decided I can (*check one*):

☐ Get copies of my most recent cholesterol readings.

☐ Write my total cholesterol level here
_____ mg/dl (date: _____).

☐ Write my HDL cholesterol level here _____ mg/dl
(date: _____).

☐ Write my LDL cholesterol level here _____ mg/dl
(date: _____).

☐ Write my triglyceride level here _____ mg/dl
(date: _____).

☐ Ask my health care provider about having a lipid panel taken or
get a BioSafe Cholesterol Panel at the pharmacy, so I can take it
at home (or call 847-234-8111 or visit www.ebiosafe.com).

☐ Contact my hospital or pharmacy to see when they have free
cholesterol screenings.

☐ Quit smoking.

☐ Drink less alcohol.

☐ Get 20 minutes of physical activity every day.

☐ Other: _____.

☺ **How fat is your blood?**

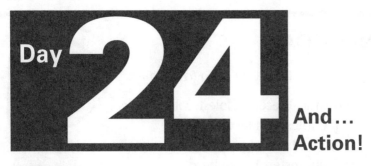

Day 24

And... Action!

 We have so many entertainment options these days that we can consider ourselves spoiled. Most homes have several TVs. Even our cars have TVs! We can sit for hours on end in front of our computers or spend days playing video games. All that screen time comes with a price. The more time we spend sitting on the couch or parked in front of the computer, the less physical activity we get, and that adds up to extra pounds. Let's look at how television viewing affects both children and adults.

Children

- About 30% of children aged 2–6 years have a TV in their room. Watching too much TV keeps kids away from healthier activities, such as family time, playing outside, and getting sleep.
- Most children under the age of 4 cannot tell the difference between a commercial and TV programming. Children as young as 2 years old see more than 20,000 television commercials a year.
- The average American child spends about 1,000 hours more time in front of the TV than in school.
- Each hour spent staring at a screen increases the risk of being overweight.
- Food and beverages advertised on TV are often high in fats, sugar, and/or salt.

Adults

- The average American adult spends about four hours a day watching television. That's about two months out of every year glued to the couch! If that's you, you're missing out on countless valuable steps.

- By the time the average American reaches age 65, nine entire years will have been spent watching TV.
- Many people enjoy snacking while watching TV.

About 50% of our population's increase in weight has been associated with watching too much TV. Cutting that time to fewer than 10 hours per week and increasing physical activity to 30 minutes a day can help prevent diabetes and prevent obesity.

PERSONAL GOAL

Today (date _____), I decided I can (*check one*):

☐ Get up and stretch at least every hour while watching the tube.

☐ Cut out 30 minutes of TV time a day.

☐ Put a treadmill or exercise equipment in front of the TV and get on it!

☐ Write down how much TV I watch and how many steps I take every day.

☐ Stop eating in front of the TV.

☐ Not watch any TV for an entire day.

☐ Other: _____.

Can I help it if I like watching cooking shows and triathlons?

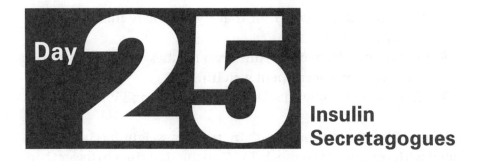

Insulin Secretagogues

Who takes this drug?

Insulin secretagogues are used in people with type 2 diabetes.

What is an insulin secretagogue?

Insulin secretagogues are a group of medications that cause the pancreas to release more insulin. Several different types are available, including combination pills.

- Amaryl (glimepiride)
- Micronase, Diabeta, or Glynase (glyburide)
- Glucotrol (glipizide)
- Prandin (repaglinide)
- Starlix (nateglinide)

How do insulin secretagogues work?

These drugs knock on the front door of the pancreas and demand that insulin come out and go into the bloodstream. If the pancreas does not have enough insulin-producing beta-cells, these medications don't help. Insulin secretagogues are often used in combination with other medications that lower glucose, such as biguanides (Glucophage), thiazolidinediones (such as Actos or Avandia), and/or long-acting insulin (such as Lantus or Levemir).

Possible side effects

Hypoglycemia with symptoms (such as irritability, shakiness, sweating, dizziness, fast heartbeat, hunger, blurred vision, weakness, drowsiness, or difficulty walking or talking).

Warning

These drugs can cause prolonged hypoglycemia (up to 72 hours) in the elderly or in those with kidney problems. Some may experience slight weight gain. The increased risk of hypoglycemia makes it important to take them with food. Alcohol should also be avoided. If you take an insulin secretagogue, be prepared to treat hypoglycemia with fast-acting glucose.

PERSONAL GOAL

Today (date _____), I decided I can (*check one*):

☐ Carry 15 grams of fast-acting glucose with me at all times (three glucose tablets, a small box of raisins, a small juice box, or a small tube of frosting).

☐ Limit alcohol if I am taking an insulin secretagogue.

☐ Report unexplained lows to my doctor.

☐ Tell my doctor why I haven't been taking my medication, regardless of the reason (e.g., don't like how I feel on the drug, expense, side effects).

☐ Ask my health care provider to suggest another medication if my blood glucose levels are still high on these drugs.

☐ Other: _____.

Insulin secretagogues are not places of worship.

Day 26

Coffee and Cigarettes

Cup of joe

Enjoying a cup of coffee is perfectly fine as long as you don't add a ton of sugar and cream. If you don't know the nutrient contents of your favorite coffee drinks, prepare yourself. Some of those specialty drinks have the same amount of calories, fat, and carbohydrates as a fast-food meal. Know what you are consuming. Know how your coffee choices affect you and your diabetes.

What about tea? Aside from caffeine (tea generally has less caffeine than coffee or soda) and cream-and-sugar issues, tea provides many health benefits and does not pose a problem for people with diabetes.

Smoking: it gets in more than just your eyes.

Would you be outraged if someone slipped a drug into your bloodstream without your permission? Nonsmokers, beware! This happens every time you take in a breath of secondhand smoke. Walk around most outdoor public areas and you'll likely encounter plumes of cigarette smoke from people mingling in corridors or hovering around entranceways. You're breathing in toxins. So much for trying to get out for some fresh air!

What can you do? Be on the lookout for cigarette smoke and try to avoid it. Short of holding your breath, make a plan to get away from it. What if your partner smokes? Decide what you are willing to accept and negotiate the rest. Your health is on the line. It's one thing if someone else decides to smoke—it's their body—but it's quite a different issue if they turn you into a passive smoker.

What a drag. For years, the Surgeon General has said that smoking is hazardous to your health. As obvious as that sounds, many smokers are unaware of the basic dangers they face. People who have diabetes and smoke are 11 times more likely to have a heart attack than those who have diabetes and don't smoke.

Ready for more? Smoking increases the risks for blindness, kidney disease, impotence, amputation, tooth loss (over 40% of people over age 65 who smoke lose their teeth), bad breath, and facial wrinkling. Same goes for cigar and pipe smokers. If that's not enough, think about what nicotine exposure does to a fetus or newborn: it increases the chances for obesity and diabetes later in life.

Ready to put out the fire? Quitting smoking is not easy, but researchers have found a method that works well.

1. Make a list of reasons why you want to quit (e.g., for your health, your kids, save hundreds of dollars).
2. Pick a quitting date and stick to it. Plan how you will fight the urge to smoke (e.g., go for a walk, go out a different door, don't hang out with smokers). Ask your health care provider to recommend a prescription (combining the nicotine patch with the drug Zyban is nearly 90% effective).
3. Change your habits. If you smoke on the porch in a nice comfortable chair, smoke standing up. Don't smoke while driving (have a smoke-free car). Smoke alone (it's not as fun as smoking with the gang). Figure out what triggers your desire for a cigarette.
4. Prepare your environment to quit. Get rid of ashtrays and lighters. Wash your clothes, so they don't smell like smoke. Buy only a single pack at a time, not a carton. Tap into a support system (many hospitals offer free smoking-cessation classes). Ask your smoking pals to not offer you cigarettes.

PERSONAL GOAL

Today (date _____), I decided I can (*check one*):

☐ Find out how many carbohydrates and calories are in my favorite cappuccino, latte, or specialty coffee drink.

☐ Avoid secondhand smoke.

☐ Pick a day to quit smoking.

☐ Request help from my health care provider, so I can kick the habit.

☐ Get help quitting smoking by calling 1-800-NO-BUTTS or 1-800-QUIT-NOW.

☐ Calculate how much money I'll save by cutting out lattes or cigarettes.

☐ Other: _____.

Make me a secondhand smoker only if I can make you a secondhand diabetic.

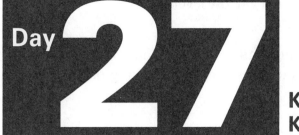

Day 27

Kidney Kindness

Wouldn't I know if something was wrong with my kidneys?

Not necessarily. Early kidney disease typically has no symptoms. Late stages of kidney disease can be accompanied by swelling, weight gain due to fluid retention, poor appetite, fatigue, headache, itchiness, and very little urine output. Prevention is very important because it is very difficult to reverse kidney disease. The longer you have diabetes, the higher your risk for kidney problems; that's why you want to prevent problems in the first place.

Lean, mean, filtering machines

Your kidneys are like super vacuum cleaners that remove toxins and waste from the blood. Each kidney has more than a million tiny blood vessels called nephrons that continuously filter blood. All of the blood in your body passes through the kidneys about 20 times every hour. The kidneys remove water and waste and get rid of it by creating urine. They also return the water that has been filtrated back into the bloodstream, thus maintaining the body's water balance.

What are my chances of having kidney problems?

Recent studies suggest that about 20% of people with diabetes develop kidney disease (also called nephropathy). Although all people with diabetes are at risk, some factors are associated with an increased risk of developing nephropathy:

- Certain ethnicities, especially African Americans, Asian Americans, Mexican Americans, and Native Americans.
- Smoking.

- Long-term high blood glucose levels.
- High blood pressure.

You can't change your family, but you can do things to change your blood glucose, blood pressure, and smoking habit (if you've got one).

Get microalbumin and creatinine urine tests!

A simple urine test checks your kidney health by measuring the amount of protein (small amounts of protein are called microalbumin) and creatinine (a component of blood filtered into the urine) to determine your risk for kidney problems. It is recommended that people have this test done once a year because it is the strongest method of detecting future kidney and cardiovascular disease.

Kidney care

With the kidneys, you don't want to wait for something to go wrong. Protect them! Here are some ways to protect your kidneys.

- Keep blood glucose in the target range as much as possible.
- Control blood pressure to less than 130/80 mmHg.
- Stop smoking!
- Ask a dietitian about kidney-friendly food choices (protein and water restriction may be necessary).
- Stay hydrated, if your doctor says your kidneys can handle it. Drinking plenty of water helps your kidneys function properly, just like changing the oil in your car helps it run efficiently.
- Have blood tests performed to check the overall function of your kidneys, including the blood urea nitrogen (BUN) test and creatinine test.
- Exercise regularly.
- Maintain a healthy weight.
- Discuss other medications you are taking with your physician or pharmacist.

When bad things happen to good kidneys, the goal is to minimize further damage. Hypoglycemia can occur if the kidneys begin to lose their ability to filter out insulin. Other signs of worsening kidney disease include escalating blood pressure, increased potassium levels (hyperkalemia), and anemia (low blood count).

Imagine what your home would look like if you couldn't take the garbage out ever again. For kidneys that have failed, dialysis is like an arrangement to have the trash removed by other people. No one wants dialysis. That would be like wanting a root canal, but it's a vital and necessary procedure if you want to continue living life to its fullest.

PERSONAL GOAL

Today (date _____), I decided I can (*check one*):

☐ Ask to have the microalbumin and creatinine tests done (and get a copy of the results).

☐ Ask to have the BUN and creatinine blood tests done (and yes, get copies of the results).

☐ Report any problems with my urine right away (e.g., pain, burning, urgency, frequency, difficulty urinating, blood or pus in the urine).

☐ Quit smoking.

☐ Avoid all sources of secondhand smoke.

☐ Drink one more glass of water every day.

☐ Check with my doctor to see if I need to restrict my protein intake (see a dietitian for a specialized plan).

☐ Bring all of my medications to my pharmacist to ask if any are tough on my kidneys.

☐ Other: _____.

Don't kid around with my kidneys.

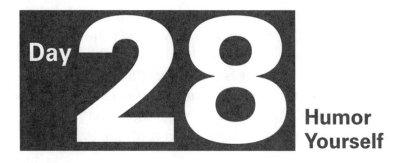

Day

28

Humor Yourself

 Diabetes is no laughing matter, yet laughing can help people manage their diabetes. Some studies have shown that laughing can lower blood glucose levels, but what's funny about diabetes?

The stigma of diabetes is often portrayed negatively, and attention focuses only on the seriousness of the disease. Moreover, dealing with all of the self-care management issues on a day-by-day basis can be overwhelming. You may not think that humor can be a great defense against diabetes, but there's always room to learn and here's why.

Humor...

- Increases endorphins, lowers anxiety, and lowers blood pressure.
- Reduces stress and burnout and reduces pain.
- Allows for the expression of anger. Language was invented because we need to communicate. Humor was invented as a way to complain. Listen to any comedian: they are complaining! Dealing with a chronic disease can trigger anger, and humor is a wonderful way to process those emotions.
- Improves learning. Those "ha, ha" moments turn into "aha" moments.
- Improves immune function.
- Is used as a weight-loss therapy.
- Is a low-carb source of energy.

Humor is required for everyone's health. More research on humor therapy has occurred in the past 40 years than ever before. We now know you don't have to laugh *at* something in order to reap the benefits of a good, healthy chuckle. You just have to laugh. There are about 1,000 worldwide laugh clubs that meet to laugh. These laugh clubs get a group of people together and just start laughing. Next thing you know, you're laughing at someone's laugh. It feels great afterwards, as strange as this may sound.

Finding Your Funny Bone

1. Be on the lookout for humor—it's everywhere. How many times do we pass funny signs and humorous situations but don't recognize them because we're taking our lives too seriously? Take a deep breath, look around yourself, and realize that life is funny, if you're paying attention to it.
2. Allow yourself to be silly. This doesn't happen overnight. You have to take risks. But be careful not to do or say anything that might be considered offensive.
3. Learn what amuses you. Did you know cartoons are the most universally accepted form of humor?
4. Learn to laugh at yourself.

By shifting your perspective to the lighter side of the health-disease continuum, you can gain the confidence needed to successfully live and manage your diabetes. Who needs more gloom and doom? Search for humor; it is therapeutic, whether or not it has to do with your diabetes. Your life is much bigger than a disease.

You rarely hear people exclaim, "I'm so thrilled I have diabetes!" Yet it's not uncommon to hear "Diabetes was the best thing that happened to me—I got my health in order." That is certainly not everyone's perspective. Diabetes does take a lot of work, and humor can help you take it in stride. The key to humor is within your reach at all times; you only need to remember to grab that key and use it.

PERSONAL GOAL

Today (date _____), I decided I can (*check one*):

☐ Find at least one funny thing today.
☐ Smile at the next person I see.
☐ Laugh at myself in the mirror tomorrow morning.
☐ Accept the diagnosis, but not the negatively-portrayed prognosis of diabetes.
☐ Commit to focusing on the positive.
☐ Go back to my TV and watch something funny.
☐ Walk to a comedy club.
☐ Look for funny titles or names in the paper.
☐ Reach beyond myself and do something goofy and out of character.
☐ Check out the Pet Pancreas humorous talking keychain at www.tgarnero.com.
☐ Other: _____.

Diabetes means I have a license to be a finicky eater.

WEEK 4: REVIEW

Today's date: _____

You have conquered one month of learning about diabetes self-management. Without boarding this train, you wouldn't advance to the next station in life. You've taken that step and are on your way!

Please list the following in looking back over your first 30 days:

Before meal readings average_____ mg/dl
2 hours after meal readings_____ mg/dl
(Before meal target is 70–130 mg/dl; 2 hours after meals is less than 180 mg/dl. It takes time to get there.)

Last blood pressure reading _____ mmHg
(target is less than 130/80 mmHg)

What was your highest glucose?_____ Lowest? _____
Do you know why?

Favorite meal where your glucose went up less than 50 points _____

What type of exercise did you do this past week?
_____For how long? _____

Do you feel better equipped to deal with your diabetes diagnosis? Why or why not? _____
_____

Did you take your medication on time?
Circle one: Nearly always   Sometimes   Almost never

Did you take care of your teeth and gums? _____
_____

Are you committed to allowing more humor into your life?
_____

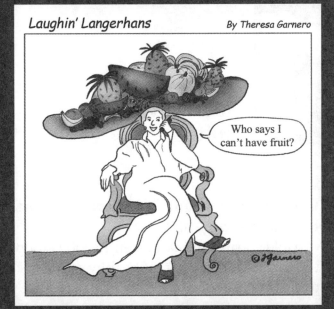

Laughin' Langerhans   By Theresa Garnero

Who says I can't have fruit?

Month

2

Week 1

Flourish with Fruit

I was told to cut out fruit because it makes my blood sugar go up.

Who told you to eliminate an entire food group? Science proves that fruits are an integral part of healthy eating. Like all other food groups that contain carbohydrate, fruits can raise your glucose level. They pack a carb punch, so you need to know how much to eat so you don't go overboard. You don't need to be a nutritionist to figure this out, but you do need to give it some thought because fruit doesn't come with a nutrition facts label.

Serving size is the key. Do you enjoy a whole bowl of cherries or tall glasses of orange juice? How about huge fruit smoothies from the health food store? Making choices like these can send your blood glucose into outer space. Think about how many oranges are needed to get four ounces of juice. You'll end up with the sugar content of several oranges just from one glass. Shoot for a serving size that you can visualize filling a cupped hand. Current recommendations suggest that people should eat one or two cups of fruit a day and not all at once.

Maybe loving fruit isn't your problem. Nearly four out of every five of adults do not eat as much fruit as they should. If you don't eat any fruit at all, try to invite nature's candy into your diet. Go for simplicity. Start with one serving of fruit two or three days a week and build up from there.

Is fruit a good snack choice?

Yes! Choose from fresh, frozen, canned (but check the sugar content first; go for light syrup, packed in its own juice or water), or dried fruit. If you drink juice, try diluting it with water.

What's a serving size of fruit?

Choose one small fruit; 1/2 cup of fresh, canned, or frozen fruit; 1/4 cup dried fruit; or 4 oz of juice.

EAT YOUR VEGGIES

Cup both hands in front of you. That's the recommended portion size for salad or uncooked vegetables (1 cup); the largest serving size of any food group. For cooked veggies, the serving size is 1/2 a cup. Every day, we need to eat at least 1 1/2 cups of veggies, but 70% of us do not. Veggies are low in calories, low in sugar, and high in fiber.

What was the last veggie you ate and when? How was it prepared? Most of us turn our noses up when it comes to choosing vegetables on a regular basis. For people with diabetes, for people trying to lower cholesterol or blood pressure, and for folks who want to lose weight, vegetables can be the ticket to health. Eat plenty of dark-green vegetables such as broccoli, spinach, and other dark, leafy greens. Orange is okay when it comes to choices like carrots and sweet potatoes. How about giving your veggies a little extra punch with vegetable broth and dried spices (oregano or Italian seasonings)? There are so many fun, flavorful veggies out there. If you don't like one, try another, and another, and another.

What is a starchy vegetable?

Starchy veggies are those that contain more carbohydrate, such as peas, corn, potatoes, yams, and sweet potatoes.

What's the serving size of vegetables?

Choose at least 1 cup of fresh vegetables or 1/2 cup cooked vegetables. Only 8% of people eat the recommended amount of fruits and veggies. Today, let's turn that dismal statistic around, one serving of fruit and veggies at a time.

If you just can't get started on bringing vegetables into your life, think about it this way. Eating water-rich, low-fat foods like fruits and veggies encourages weight loss. These low-calorie dense foods can make you feel more full, so you'll eat less!

PERSONAL GOAL

This week (date _____), I decided I can (*check one*):

☐ Keep a bag of frozen veggies at work and home and have 1 cup of veggies at lunch.
☐ Eat fruit rather than drink it.
☐ Have a small fruit as a snack (the size of my cupped hand).
☐ Try a new fruit.
☐ Have a fruit choice with lunch.
☐ Try a new vegetable.
☐ Start adding a serving of vegetables to dinner two to three days a week and work up to covering half of my plate with veggies at every meal.
☐ Help out my sweet tooth by giving it fruit rather than candy.

**Veggies are my friends.
I should see them more often.**

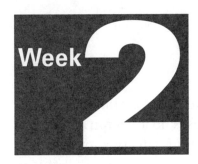

Week 2

Glucose Bumps in the Road

Blood pressure

Higher fasting blood glucose levels arise more often in people with high blood pressure than in those with normal blood pressure. No one really knows why this connection exists, but it does. So, if you have hypertension, be sure to get help in treating it.

Dawn phenomenon

This has nothing to do with daylight savings time; it's about the time of day it occurs. The dawn phenomenon is the body's response to hormones released in the early morning hours. This occurs for everyone. When we sleep, hormones are released to help maintain and restore cells within our bodies. These hormones cause blood glucose levels to rise. For people with diabetes who do not have enough circulating insulin to keep this increase of glucose under control, the end result is higher glucose readings in the morning.

If you find that you are experiencing the dawn phenomenon, try exercising later in the day. This may help a bit. Talk with your health care provider about possibly adjusting your medications. Regardless, be sure to eat breakfast every day, because doing so tells your body to turn off these problematic hormones.

Exercise

Right after exercise, you may see a temporary increase in glucose values. This happens because the liver releases its stored glucose to help your muscles keep working. Do not get discouraged if you see slight blood glucose elevation after a workout. Your numbers over the next 24 hours will be in a better range than if you hadn't exercised. Also, be on the lookout for lows several hours after finishing exercising. This is when the liver takes glucose out of the blood-stream to replenish its glucose storage.

Medication effectiveness

When your blood glucose levels come into the target range, a unique problem can arise. Because your pancreas is no longer in a toxic environment, your medication becomes more effective, which puts you at greater risk for blood glucose lows. If you think that this is happening to you, call your health care provider. He or she may want to lower your medication dosage.

Overtreating lows

If you have personally experienced a low, you know the panic feeling that accompanies it. One gentleman reported he treated his lows by sticking his head in the fridge (with his fanny sticking out—nice visual), and eating everything in sight. Overtreating lows can cause hyperglycemia and increase calories and thus, weight gain. What about having a hypoglycemia kit (with 15 grams of glucose, and a snack to eat afterwards)?

Steroids

If you have ever suffered from bursitis, arthritis, or other inflammatory issues and received a shot of cortisone or other steroid treatment, you know how helpful steroids are. But they can also raise blood glucose levels for up to three days after receiving treatment.

Stress and illness

Stress has negative effects on the body and can raise blood glucose levels. Stress can also arise in seemingly happy occasions: vacation, travel, weddings, family gatherings, retirement, and winning the lottery. If you get a high number that just doesn't make sense, take a step back and examine your stress level. Search out ways to reduce and cope with the stress in your life. Illness can also raise your glucose levels. Stick with frequent testing whenever you do not feel well.

Somogyi effect

The Somogyi effect, also known as rebound hyperglycemia, is a pattern of undetected blood glucose lows followed by highs (hyperglycemia). Typically, this happens in the middle of the night but can also occur when too much insulin is circulating. The Somogyi effect is caused when insulin or diabetes pills work too well at the wrong time and send blood glucose levels way down. To counteract this imbalance, the liver releases its stored glucose. The end result is that blood glucose levels can swing too high in the other direction.

If you are waking up with high blood glucose readings and are wondering if you're experiencing the Somogyi effect, try checking your blood glucose levels in the middle of the night to see if you are low. Try setting your alarm between 2 and 3 a.m. so you can wake up to check your blood glucose. The best way to correct the Somogyi effect is to prevent it from happening in the first place. It takes detective work to figure out what made the glucose plummet. Is it too much medication? Not enough bedtime snack? Try a time-released glucose bar (ask your pharmacist where to find one) or a hearty bedtime snack (piece of toast with peanut butter, some cottage cheese, yogurt, or some nuts and a small piece of cheese), but check with your health care team first to see if this is an appropriate way to counteract the Somogyi effect.

ACTIVITY INVENTORY

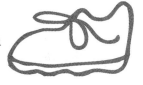

Nearly 80% of insulin resistance happens in the skeletal muscles. This means if you work your muscles regularly through exercise, you will use insulin more efficiently and change the course of this disease. If you reduce your insulin resistance, your pancreas won't have to work so hard to make extra insulin.

Are you willing to make an investment in your body with some form of dedicated exercise almost every day? What can you do today?

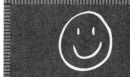

My pancreas is smiling—I took a 30-minute brisk walk.

PERSONAL GOAL

This week (date _____), I decided I can (*check one*):

☐ Have a hearty bedtime snack (piece of toast with peanut butter, cottage cheese, or yogurt or some nuts and a small piece of cheese).
☐ Set the alarm for 2–3 a.m. and check my glucose.
☐ Buy glucose tablets to keep with me at all times.
☐ Check my glucose whenever I feel odd.
☐ Eat breakfast most days of the week.
☐ Test my glucose at least every four hours when I'm sick.
☐ Check glucose patterns the day after I exercise.
☐ Other: _____.

Even a psychic couldn't explain my wacky glucose readings.

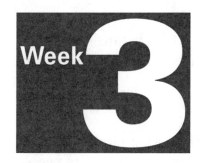

Week 3

Thiazolidinediones (TZDs)

Who takes this drug?
Thiazolidinediones (TZDs) are prescribed for people with type 2 diabetes.

What are TZDs?
TZDs help the body overcome the insulin resistance associated with type 2 diabetes, a condition in which the body's response to insulin is impaired. The two main TZDs are

- Actos (brand name) or pioglitazone (generic). The minimum dose is 15 mg a day, with a maximum of 45 mg a day. Actos also has cholesterol-lowering effects. Must be used cautiously in people with congestive heart failure.
- Avandia (brand name) or rosiglitazone (generic). The minimum dose is 4 mg a day, with a maximum of 8 mg a day. Avandia may be associated with an increased risk of heart attacks and should not be prescribed for people on insulin or on nitrates.

TZDs may be used alone or in combination with other diabetes medications, including insulin.

How do TZDs work?
TZDs decrease insulin resistance. More specifically, TZDs help cells respond to the insulin that is present in the body. It may take four to eight weeks of consistent treatment before TZDs make a visible change in blood glucose levels. TZDs are known to preserve beta-cell function.

Possible side effects

Swelling and weight gain are possible, as is liver failure. People who are prescribed TZDs should have their liver function tested before starting these drugs.

Warning

If you have a liver problem or drink excessive amounts of alcohol, TZDs are *not* for you. They should also be used cautiously in people with congestive heart failure. Be sure to report any sudden swelling or weight gain to your doctor.

PERSONAL GOAL

This week (date _____), I decided I can (*check one*):

☐ Ask for copies of my most recent liver function tests (copies of blood work).
☐ Continue to take my TZD if my blood glucose is in target range, unless advised otherwise.
☐ Take my TZD as prescribed.
☐ Tell my doctor why I haven't been taking my medication, regardless of the reason (don't like how I feel, the expense, the side effects, etc.).
☐ Call my doctor to report any swelling in my feet or ankles or if I have changes in vision.
☐ Other: _____.

 Do they charge for these pills by the letter?

Socked Away

 Foot safety is one of the most important things to consider if you have diabetes. You hear a lot of people complain about ugly therapeutic shoes, but how many of them ever talk about their choice of socks? Start at the beginning, with your socks, and treat your feet right.

What are the best kinds of socks?

Cotton socks are comfortable but tend to retain moisture close to the skin, which can make your feet sweat. Sweaty feet can lead to blisters and worse. Now there are cotton-synthetic blends that pull moisture away from the feet and can prevent blisters. Synthetic fibers include acrylic, Duraspun, ionized copper, Lycra, nylon, polyester, and X-Static.

What Should I Look For When Buying Socks?

- Cotton-synthetic blends for exercising.
- Seamless socks for leisure time (material is less important).
- For dressy occasions, limit the use of nylons and consider microfiber acrylic alternatives instead.
- Check the fabric content.
- Avoid constricting bands.
- Look for wide-fit socks if you have swollen ankles.
- Your local pharmacy may carry specialty socks. You can also visit these stores on the web:
  —Smooth Toe [www.smoothtoe-socks.com; 507-251-6092]
  —The Diabetic Sock Store [www.diabeticsockstore.com; 866-848-9327]
  —Foot Smart [www.footsmart.com; 800-707-9928]

PERSONAL GOAL

This week (date _____), I decided I can (*check one*):

☐ Check my local comprehensive pharmacy for diabetes socks.
☐ Visit websites that carry safe socks.
☐ Take a sock inventory: out with the risky ones, in with the safe ones.
☐ Ask for stylish diabetic socks for a gift.
☐ Trash my holey socks.
☐ Avoid buying socks that might cause foot problems.
☐ Discard knee-high nylons that fall down (they can bunch up and create blisters).
☐ Invest in my feet through good-fitting socks.
☐ Other: _____.

 Now I need to diversify my sock options.

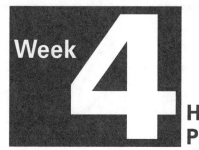

Week 4

Home Blood Pressure Monitoring

Why do I need to check my blood pressure at home?
You can minimize your risk of future problems by knowing what your blood pressure is now and acting on those numbers. By checking at home, you'll have more information to work with than just an occasional check on your visits to your doctor.

What type of monitor is best?

The manual blood pressure devices used in medical facilities are most accurate but require some training for use. For home use, select one with an inflatable cuff that goes over the arm or wrist. Highly rated home blood pressure monitors are made by Omron (www.omronhealthcare.com), microlife (www.microlifeusa.com), and Lifesource (www.andonline.com). Ask your pharmacist to point one out or order one for you.

When should I check my blood pressure?

Check it regularly. Start off by checking first thing in the morning for a week. The next week, test at another time that is convenient, like after dinner. Ask your health care provider what he or she feels would be the best time to test. Definitely check your blood pressure if you feel any heart-related symptoms, such as skipped beats, shortness of breath, chest pain or pressure, dizziness, and nausea.

Get your health care provider involved.

You need to know how to properly use the device. If the cuff is not placed correctly, results can vary widely. Have one of your health care team members watch you check your blood pressure and give you tips on how to do it the right way.

PERSONAL GOAL

This week (date _____), I decided I can (*check one*):

☐ Look for a high-quality home blood pressure monitor.

☐ Bring my home blood pressure monitor to my next medical appointment to make sure my technique is correct.

☐ Have my health care provider check the accuracy of my home blood pressure monitoring device.

☐ Check my blood pressure once a day.

☐ Write down my readings.

☐ Write down any comments about what I think might be influencing my readings (stress, late with medication, too much salt, too little exercise, too much exercise, etc.).

☐ Check my blood pressure if I have chest pain, dizziness, sore neck or jaw, numbness in the arm, unexplained sweating, or nausea.

☐ Bring my list of blood pressure readings to my next medical appointment and ask for the best plan to improve my blood pressure.

☐ Other: _____.

 My blood pressure monitor said "Uh oh" all week.

MONTH 2: REVIEW

Today's date: _____

Congratulations on making it through two months of intensive diabetes self-management. Take a minute to reflect and rate your progress.

Please circle the answer that best represents your assessment of the past two months:

CHECK NUMBERS
1. I tested my glucose:
   a. Rarely (less than 20%)
   b. Sometimes (20–80%)
   c. Mostly (more than 80%)

AVOID PROBLEMS
2. I know to call my health care provider when my glucose values are consistently above 250 mg/dl for two consecutive days or less than 70 mg/dl on any given day.
   a. Yes
   b. No

EAT WISELY
3. I have found enjoyable foods that my diabetes can handle.
   a. Yes
   b. No

BE ACTIVE
4. I am active for at least 20 minutes five days a week.
   a. Rarely (less than 20%)
   b. Sometimes (20–80%)
   c. Mostly (more than 80%)

REDUCE STRESS

5. I have tried and found new ways to deal with stress.

a. Yes

b. No

UNDERSTAND MEDICATIONS

6. I know how my medication functions.

a. Yes

b. No

REDUCE RISKS

7. I saw the dentist, or the podiatrist, or had my kidneys checked, or flossed my teeth regularly, or got a flu shot (just one of these).

a. Yes

b. No

ADD HUMOR

8. I have begun to notice the subtle humor in situations.

a. Yes

b. No

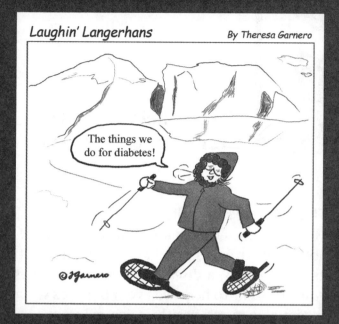

Month

3

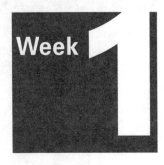

Carb-o-licious: Milk, Grains, and Desserts

The miracles of milk
Milk is highly regarded for its calcium content. And why not? Calcium helps build and maintain healthy bones and prevents osteoporosis, a disease in which the bones become fragile and easily broken. To help keep your bones as strong as they can be, it is essential to have a healthy calcium intake.

Milk also has eight other essential nutrients to keep your body energized. Besides calcium, milk contains vitamin D (which helps the body properly use its calcium and encourages absorption of other essential minerals), riboflavin (a B-vitamin that helps convert food into energy), and others, including phosphorus, protein, vitamin B12, potassium, niacin, and vitamin A. It's time for a glass of milk!

The challenge for people with diabetes, who have the same risk for osteoporosis as people without diabetes, is that milk is counted as a carb.

How much milk should I have?
The recommendation is to have two to three servings from the milk group per day. This includes eight ounces of nonfat or low-fat milk (or plain soy milk or powdered milk) or nonfat yogurt (plain or flavored, with an artificial, non-nutritive sweetener).

What if I don't drink milk? How do I get my calcium?
If you don't drink milk or eat yogurt, other food sources of calcium are low-fat cheese (1 1/2 to 2 oz is the equivalent of an 8-oz glass of milk), calcium-enriched orange juice, and milk substitutes, such as soy, rice, or almond milks. If none of these appeals to you, then taking a calcium supplement is the way to go. Make sure your calcium

supplement also includes vitamin D. Take no more than 500 mg at a time, and current research suggests that taking the supplements in the afternoon offers the best absorption. If you take both calcium and iron supplements, take them at different times.

PASTA, RICE, AND GRAINS—OH MY!

The carbohydrate group that consists of grains, cereal, rice, and pasta creates the most interest and confusion in people. Start by casting your vote for your best carb candidate. I don't like to tell people how to decide, but in this case, go for whole grains whenever they're available. Choose whole-wheat bread (look at the label to be sure this is the first ingredient), whole-wheat flour, brown or wild rice, rolled oats, and high-fiber cereals. Does that mean you can never have white rice, white pasta, or white bread? No, but you are missing out on essential nutrients—like most of the B-vitamins—when you choose refined, white carbohydrates over whole grains.

SWEET TOOTH

How did so many of us develop a sweet tooth? It is without a doubt that we love to have our sweets and that we're eating more than our share. The problem is that those sweets often contain quite a bit of carbohydrate, which spells trouble for those who want to watch their blood glucose levels.

BUYER BEWARE:
GLYCEMIC INDEX AND NET CARBS

So, what's this glycemic index thing?

You've likely heard of the glycemic index and seen it advertised on products. But what exactly is the glycemic index? Put simply, it measures the body's response to 50 grams of carbohydrate from one kind of food. Sounds helpful, right?

The issue with the glycemic index is that it *does not* measure how rapidly blood glucose levels peak, only how long the glucose will stay in the system. This seems useful, but when was the last time you ate only 50 grams of carbohydrate from one food type? Furthermore, different foods affect different people in different ways.

Tackle that Sweet Tooth

- First things first: acknowledge your sweet tooth.
- Make yourself walk to the store to buy treats and don't keep a stash in the house!
- Cut back on other carbohydrates within the meal to make an even trade for your dessert carbohydrates (avoid doing this every day).
- Seek quality, not quantity. If you are craving something in particular, don't compromise. You'll end up eating other things without satisfying the beast.
- Out of sight, out of mind. Reduce your portion sizes (don't go for that gargantuan slice of cake); ask for child-sized servings instead.
- Have fruit rather than candy.
- Check the calorie and saturated-fat content of your treats.
- Have a glass of water before you start with the dessert (water quenches thirst, not hunger). Doing this makes sure you're not eating when you're actually thirsty.
- Watch out for items labeled "sugar free." By definition, that means the item has less than a 1/2 gram of sugar or sucrose in a serving, but it will often contain as many carbohydrates (or more) than the regular product.
- Write down how much you're spending on sweets each week. Sticker shock might scare away that spendthrift sweet tooth!

There is no concrete way to say that food A will affect person A the same way as it'll affect person B.

The glycemic index can also be very misleading. For example, potatoes have a higher glycemic index than pizza. However, pizza has many more carbohydrates per serving than do potatoes. In the end, you'll get a much higher glucose effect from eating pizza than potatoes, but you wouldn't know that just by looking at the glycemic index. If you're still not confused, consider this: soft drinks and chocolate candy have a medium glycemic index!

Next time you're choosing carbohydrates, don't sweat the glycemic index. Instead, choose wisely by eating a *variety* of carbohydrates and keeping them consistent in your diet. Focus on the total carbohydrates you're taking in with each meal.

What's a net carb?

Some advertising genius thought up the concept of "net carbs" (or "carb impact") because it sells. If you doubt it, just check out the "diabetic food" section at your local grocery store. You think you are getting a product low in carbohydrate, but that's not necessarily true. The idea behind net carbs is to subtract the grams of fiber and sugar alcohols from the grams of total carbohydrate to give you the net carbs or glycemic load. But you need a high-fiber food (with more than 5 grams) for this formula to work and not all foods are high in fiber. Also, many people underestimate portion sizes and end up eating too large a portion of the food to make its net carbs matter. For the time being, you're better off leaving net carbs on the shelf.

PERSONAL GOAL

This week (date _____), I decided I can (*check one*):

☐ Satisfy my sweet tooth and get calcium with low-fat chocolate milk.
☐ Pick milk over soda at lunch.
☐ Share my dessert.
☐ Check the label on bread for carbohydrate and fiber content and to see if it is whole grain.
☐ Choose high-fiber cereals with milk for my breakfasts (or snacks).
☐ For that sweet tooth, cut down on junk food and pick just one sweet treat a day.
☐ Other: _____.

☺ **They do make small potato chip bags—you just have to buy them in bulk.**

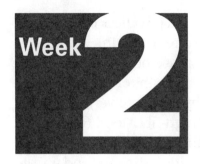

Week 2

Fun in Function

For those of you who are exercising regularly—and for those of you who aren't—check out these ideas for inspiring physical activity. Circle at least two that you are willing to do this month.

- Walk around a park I've never visited.
- See a new exhibit in a museum.
- See how many different kinds of birds I can spot in a 30-minute walk.
- Go bowling.
- Plant something.
- Go rollerblading.
- Take a bike ride through a scenic route.
- Buy and use a hula hoop or jump rope.
- Play golf (regular or miniature).
- Join an ultimate Frisbee league.
- Take a dance class.
- Find an exercise pal to take the "work" out of "workout."
- Walk to your next dinner date.
- Do nude yoga.
- Stretch to *Swan Lake*.
- Walk somewhere for a picnic.
- Saunter downtown to people watch.
- Do jumping jacks in the pool.
- Tread water.

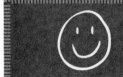 **Forget about fun. I exercise so I can eat!**

Meter Accuracy

How do I know my meter is accurate?

It's common to second guess your meter's accuracy when a glucose result doesn't make sense. Even though today's glucose meters are leaps and bounds better than the old methods (urine test strips), a variety of factors can affect the accuracy of a glucose meter. Here is a short list of possible explanations for an unexpected reading.

Measure My Meter

- The calibration of the meter may be off (call the manufacturer)
- Low batteries
- Old or expired test strips
- Third-party (generic) test strips
- Temperature and humidity (extreme heat or cold can affect readings)
- Altitude
- Size of blood sample (don't oversqueeze your finger to get enough blood for a sample)
- The amount of red blood cells in the blood (or hematocrit level): anemia, sickle cell anemia, and kidney failure can affect hematocrit levels
- Dirty hands
- Dirt on the meter
- Severe dehydration can result in false high readings
- Alternative site testing (sites other than the fingertips can have differing glucose levels)

Check your meter once a month.

Some manufacturers include a glucose control solution (water with a controlled amount of sugar) with their meters. To test the accuracy of your meter, place a drop of the glucose control solution on a test strip and insert the strip in the meter. In the instructions or on the bottle of control solution, there will be a range of glucose values. Simply see if the reading on your meter matches the range listed for the control solution. If it does, then your meter is working fine. If not, call the meter company. Check your meter's accuracy whenever you open a new package of strips or if anything happened to your meter to make you wonder if it is still working correctly (like if you dropped it down three flights of stairs).

Involve your health care provider.

Bring your meter and readings to your health care provider. If you do not have a meter, ask for help in selecting the best one. If you have one and don't like it, ask about other options.

PERSONAL GOAL

This week (date _____), I decided I can (*check one*):

☐ Call the toll-free number on the back of the meter to ask any questions and for troubleshooting help.
☐ Run a quality control test on my meter.
☐ Keep the meter and strips away from extreme temperatures.
☐ Check the expiration date on the test strips.
☐ If applicable, enter the calibration code from the outside of the strip bottle each time I open a new package of strips.
☐ Make sure my hands are clean.
☐ Turn up my lancet depth if I'm having trouble getting enough blood.
☐ Completely insert the test strip in the meter.

This call may be monitored for quality glucose control.

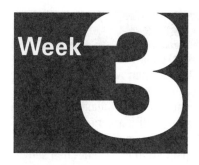

Week 3

Blood Pressure Medications

Diabetes and high blood pressure are siblings fighting for your attention. If your blood pressure is above 130/80 mmHg, you are at risk for cardiovascular complications (the big ones: heart attack and stroke). Taking blood pressure medications can extend your lease on life. People rarely like to take medications, but protecting your heart with these medications can definitely improve your odds of living a longer life.

Types of blood pressure medicines	Brand name (generic name)	Possible side effects or issues
Angiotensin-Converting Enzyme (ACE) Inhibitors (lowers blood pressure, reduces insulin resistance, protects the lining of blood vessels and kidneys; one of the first choices for treating hypertension)	**Accupril** (quinapril) **Altace** (ramipril) **Capoten** (captopril) **Mavik** (trandolapril) **Prinivil** (lisinopril) **Vasotec** (enalapril) **Zestril** (lisinopril)	May cause a cough, although that is a positive sign that the harmful chemicals that narrow blood vessels are being blocked. May aid in the prevention of diabetes and of diabetic kidney disease. A rare, but serious condition can occur with swelling in the tongue and mouth and high levels of potassium. Do not take salt substitutes or potassium without talking to a doctor. Do not use if pregnant.

Types of blood pressure medicines	Brand name (generic name)	Possible side effects or issues
Angiotensin II Receptor Blockers (ARBs) (effects are similar to those of ACE inhibitors)	**Atacand** (candesartanl) **Avapro** (irbesartan) **Cozaar** (losartan) **Diovan** (valsartan) **Micardis** (telmisartan	Blocks harmful chemicals that can narrow blood vessels without the coughing sometimes seen with ACE inhibitors. As a result, ARBs are more expensive.　May cause dizziness and upset stomach. Do not use salt substitutes or potassium without talking to a doctor. Do not use if pregnant.　May aid in the prevention of diabetic kidney disease.　Several guidelines recommend that people with diabetes who have heart or blood vessel disease, congestive heart failure, or protein in the urine be prescribed an ACE inhibitor or ARB, even though they don't have high blood pressure.
Calcium Channel Blockers (CCBs) (blocks calcium in the heart vessels, which makes the arteries relax and allows more oxygen in)	**Adalat** (nifedipine) **Cardizem** (diltiazem) **Norvasc** (amlodipine) **Plendil** (felodipine) **Procardia** (nifedipine)	May cause swelling in the hands or feet, constipation, upset stomach, or flushed skin. Call your doctor if you feel short of breath, have any swelling, or feel your heart has skipped beats.
Alpha Blockers (relaxes the heart vessels and slows down the heart)	**Cardura** (doxazosin) **Hytrin** (terazosin) **Minipress** (prazosin)	May cause sudden dizziness if you get up too fast, especially with the first few doses. Do not suddenly stop taking alpha blockers.
Beta Blockers (relaxes blood vessels and helps the heart beat regularly; also used for chest pain)	**Inderal** (propranolol) **Tenormin** (atenolol) **Toprol** (metoprolol)	Helps the heart work easier. Some risky side effects: may block your ability to detect hypoglycemia, increase insulin resistance, and worsen diabetes control. Some experience depression, nightmares, and insomnia.

Types of blood pressure medicines	Brand name (generic name)	Possible side effects or issues
Hydrochlorothia-zides (known as a water pill or thiazide diuretic; relaxes small blood vessels)	**HTCZ**	Inexpensive and used in combination with many types of blood pressure pills. For doses above 12.5 mg, some may experience cramps, rashes, and loss of potassium.
Combination: **Alpha and Beta Blockers** (see descriptions above)	**Coreg** (carvedilol)	Lowers insulin resistance. May cause sudden dizziness when standing up. May cause upset stomach and mask signs of low blood glucose.
Combination: **Renin-angiotensin-aldosterone system (RAAS)**	**Lotrel** (amlodipine and benazepril)	Has calcium channel blocker and ACE inhibitor qualities. See descriptions above.

PERSONAL GOAL

This week (date _____), I decided I can (*check one*):

☐ Tell my health care provider, certified diabetes educator, or pharmacist about any possible side effects I might be having.
☐ Call my health care provider immediately if I have any swelling of the tongue or mouth.
☐ Report swelling of the hands or ankles.
☐ Get on the phone to report shortness of breath to my doctor.
☐ Make an appointment to discuss my blood pressure medications.
☐ Let my doctor know if I've skipped or stopped taking my blood pressure pills.
☐ Pick up a home blood pressure monitor and start using it.
☐ Other: _____.

Is it a good thing to know my doctor's number by heart?

Diabetes Isn't Sexy

 Both men and women battle the issue of sex and diabetes. Although sex is so important to all of us, very few people are willing to discuss the complications that diabetes can bring into an otherwise healthy sex life. So, put aside your inhibitions and fears, and let's talk about sex.

What Kinds of Sexual Problems Are Common in People with Diabetes?

- Lack of interest/decreased libido (more common in women than in men)
- Unable to climax (about the same frequency for women and men)
- Climax too quickly (more common in men than in women)
- Physical pain (more common in women than in men)
- Not pleasurable (more common in women than in men)
- Erection issues for men (at least 1 in 4 men)
- Lubrication issues for women (at least 1 in 5 women)

About 40% of men and women avoided sex because of these problems.

"Don't ask, don't tell" in health care

Need proof we aren't talking about sexual health in the health care world? Fewer than 20% of people with diabetes who have sexual problems talk about it with their health care providers. Worse, during regular medical visits, health care providers rarely ask about sexual health.

Regardless of your sexual orientation, your health status, and your sexual life, you need to bring up sexual issues with your health care providers if you have questions and he or she isn't asking you about them first. If you find that your health care provider isn't willing to help you with your total health—including your sexual health—then it may be time to look around for a new health care provider.

How Do You Avoid or Prevent Sexual Problems?

- *Pre-pregnancy planning.* An unplanned pregnancy adds unnecessary risks for your baby. If you want children, see an endocrinologist first to check which medications to stop and if switching to insulin will be necessary (certain diabetes pills cause birth defects). It is important to maintain good blood glucose levels during pregnancy, too. Discuss which birth control approach or contraceptive devices would work best for you until you're ready to become pregnant.

- *Glycemic control.* The better your blood glucose, the better your sex life. When blood glucose levels are in the target range, you'll have more energy to waltz down lover's lane.

- *Avoid hypoglycemia.* Sex is exercise (a *fun* type), and it can cause you to go low. Like any intense workout, you want to know what your blood glucose is before you start. You may need a pre-intimacy snack!

- *Limit alcohol.* Alcohol can lead to hypoglycemia. Making love in a state of hypoglycemia can turn a tender moment into a crisis.

- *Nutrition.* Those who eat better see a positive effect on sexual ability. Count those carbohydrates if you're using whipped cream or chocolate sauce. Semen and vaginal fluids do not have carbohydrates.

- *Exercise.* Those who exercise more have an increased ability in the bedroom.

- *Check hormones.* Low testosterone levels are more common in men than in women. This can cause loss of sex drive and depression. Replacement therapy is a possible treatment.

- *Don't be in a rush.* Making love should not be an environment in which you put yourself under pressure. Take your time. Roll out the red carpet. Play sexy music. Dim those lights and get flowers. Have a romantic dinner. Use foreplay. Be intimate with caresses. Use your imagination.

- *Communicate with your partner.* Unless you are with a mind reader, the only way your loved one will know what is going on is if you talk. This is very challenging. Most people would rather avoid sex entirely than have a candid conversation, let alone find out what pleases his or her partner, including experimenting with new positions, toys, or whatever rocks your partner's world.

Special issues for men

Erectile dysfunction (ED, also called impotence) is the inability to get and maintain an erection and is the most common sexual problem for men. High levels of glucose can damage the nerves and blood vessels in the penis. When this happens, the interest in sex and the ability to perform it are two different things. Treatment for ED depends on your overall health status. Discuss treatment options with your health care provider.

Treatments for Erectile Dysfunction

- Pills (Cialis, Levitra, Viagra)
- Suppositories inserted into the tip of the penis (Muse)
- Pumps that bring blood into the penis
- Penile injections just prior to sex
- Implants
- Other medications may cause ED (e.g., blood pressure or depression pills)

Special issues for women

Uncontrolled diabetes can kill the mood for sexual relations and damage the nerves that affect vaginal lubrication. You may be interested in sex, but the dryness can cause pain. Over-the-counter personal lubricants can help. Menstrual cycles tend to send blood glucose levels higher, too. You may need more medications (for diabetes and/or pain), more exercise, or a slight reduction in carbohydrates in the diet. Conversely, during menopause, estrogen and progesterone levels drop, which contributes to dryness and may reduce the desire to have sex.

Other issues common to women with diabetes include vaginal yeast and urinary tract infections (UTIs). Yeast infections usually involve vaginal itching; a white, odorless "cheese-like" discharge; and pain with urination and sex. Yeast infections can be treated with over-the-counter medications. Also, eating low-fat yogurt with active cultures helps maintain the balance of healthy bacteria.

A UTI occurs when bacteria enters the bladder. Symptoms include a severe burning sensation during urination, the frequent urge to urinate (and only a few drops come out), foul-smelling urine, and/

or pain on one side of your back. Left untreated, this can lead to a kidney infection and body-wide infection (sepsis). To treat a UTI, you will need an oral antibiotic from your health care provider and to control blood glucose levels as much as possible (high glucose levels encourage bacteria to grow). Drink sugar-free cranberry juice to help treat and prevent UTIs. Avoid tight underwear or clothes that limit the flow of air.

PERSONAL GOAL

This week (date _____), I decided I can (*check one*):

- ☐ Tell my partner I am struggling with an issue related to sex.
- ☐ Ask to have my testosterone level tested and get copies of the results (men only).
- ☐ Report sex-related concerns to my health care provider.
- ☐ Take my time with sex.
- ☐ Buy an over-the-counter lubricant (K-Y jelly or Astroglide).
- ☐ Have a little snack before sex.
- ☐ Other: _____.

☺ **I feel sorry for all the guys named ED.**

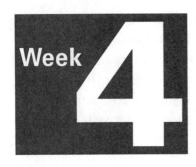

Week 4 — The Art of Travel

Is it time to recharge the batteries with a long-deserved vacation or are you headed out on a business trip? A little planning goes a long way to ensuring that diabetes doesn't interfere with your travel plans.

Before you go

If you know you are going on a long trip, you may want to get a checkup about one month before you leave. Ask your doctor about immunizations (if you are traveling abroad), how to adjust medications with time zone changes (when five or fewer time zones are crossed, no change is required, but more than that, get advice), and what to do if you get ill on your trip. Also ask for an extra prescription for diabetes medications and glucose monitoring supplies (keep these with you at all times during travel), so if your luggage is misplaced or stolen, you will have an easier time getting your diabetes supplies replaced.

What should I pack?

If you are traveling by air, you can request a diabetic meal in advance or plan on counting carbohydrates. Call the airline at least 24 hours in advance to make sure that you're able to bring your diabetes supplies on board the plane. Always carry diabetes supplies and medications in your carry-on luggage. Doing this will save your life if your luggage is lost. Also, the extreme temperatures in the luggage compartment in airplanes can damage medications.

At the airport, notify the security screener that you have diabetes and that you are carrying your supplies with you. If you have trouble getting through security, ask for a supervisor to assist you.

Don't worry about having your meter or insulin go through the X-ray. If you are wearing an insulin pump, advise the screener that it cannot be removed because it is attached to a catheter under your skin. If traveling alone, consider telling at least one person you have diabetes.

Things to Pack

- Medications (and insulin) with their original pharmacy/prescription labels. Make sure the labels match the name on your airline ticket.
- Blood glucose monitor and supplies (must have manufacturer's name on it and lancets must be capped).
- Bring twice the amount of diabetes supplies you think you might need.
- Glucose tablets, if you are at risk for going low.
- Snacks (crackers with cheese or peanut butter, protein bars, or nuts).
- Socks and shoes that won't cause blisters.
- Medical insurance cards.
- Emergency phone numbers, including your health care team.
- Medical alert bracelet, especially if you take diabetes medication or insulin.
- Insulated bag to keep insulin cool (opened insulin vials can be stored at room temperature [59–86°F]).
- Water.
- Sunscreen.

PERSONAL GOAL

This week (date _____), I decided I can (*check one*):

☐ Schedule an appointment for a checkup one month prior to leaving on a long trip.

☐ Ask my health care provider for an extra diabetes medication prescription in case I need it while traveling.

☐ Ask my doctor what to do if I become sick while traveling.

☐ Make sure the prescription label is visible on all my diabetes medications.

☐ Get a translated diabetes-medical alert card (available in many languages).

☐ Pack my diabetes kit a few days before I leave (including medications, glucose tablets, and snacks) and add my meter as I leave for the airport.

☐ Carry diabetes medicines and meter supplies with me along with my medical alert bracelet.

☐ Contact the destination to find out about the meal times and if refrigeration is available (for insulin users).

☐ Bring a list of emergency contact phone numbers and put key contact numbers in my cell phone.

☐ Write down a list of all of my medications and pack it in my carry-on luggage.

All this planning for a trip makes me want to take another vacation.

Groupies Have Lower Glucose

 Get support. Study after study has shown a strong link between having a support system and effective diabetes management.

Why?

When your support system cares for you and about your health, it is motivating. You don't feel alone and you are more likely to make positive changes in your self-care regimen if you have a strong support system. Your family and friends can play a pivotal supporting role in your diabetes care, but outside support groups can be just as (or even more) helpful.

Consider a diabetes support group.

Support groups provide opportunities for you to meet other people with diabetes in an informal atmosphere to discuss anything related to diabetes in a non-threatening environment. You can talk about the impact diabetes has on your life, ask others about their successful strategies, and get support for healthy living. It helps to be connected with someone who is in a similar situation. Often, some of the best support comes from people who are not your

What to Look For in a Support Group

- *Location*. Is transportation an issue?
- *Time*. Does the group's schedule match with yours?
- *Leader*. Who leads the group: a health care professional or someone with diabetes? Both can be very helpful and empowering, but tend to have different purposes. Which is right for you?
- *Dynamics*. Is the group's age range, culture, ethnicity, language, and/or type of diabetes a good fit for you?
- *Participation*. Do you have an opportunity to interact?
- *Perception*. Did you think your first meeting helped or not? Do you want to go back? When in doubt, give the group a second chance.

friends or family, but who specifically understand what you are going through with your diabetes.

Where can I find a diabetes support group?

You can start looking for a support group by asking your health care provider about them. You can call local hospitals and diabetes education programs to see if they have any information. You can also check with libraries and churches, and don't forget about the power of the Internet.

PERSONAL GOAL

This week (date _____), I decided I can (*check one*):

☐ Locate and attend a diabetes support group.
☐ Ask my partner to attend a class or support group with me.
☐ Talk to someone with diabetes.
☐ Talk to someone who will be supportive about my diabetes.
☐ Contact my local American Diabetes Association office at 1-800-DIABETES (1-800-342-2383) to find a local diabetes support group.
☐ Other: _____.

 My friends help me get by and get into trouble.

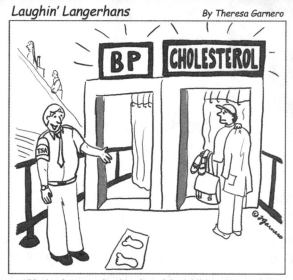

Laughin' Langerhans   By Theresa Garnero

"You've been randomly selected for additional screening."

Month

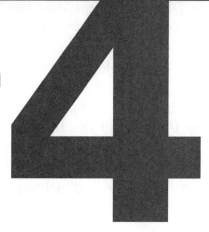

Week 1

Worth the Weight

Most adults are in a weight-loss state of mind. Our obsession with shedding pounds feeds a multibillion dollar diet industry. We'd rather spend our hard-earned dollars on fad diets, miracle supplements, packaged foods, and paid memberships to support groups than look within for the solution to losing weight. Save those dollars, because the track records for lose-weight-fast remedies are lousy, with little or no scientific research to back up their health claims. Nearly 90% of dieters, or 9 of 10 people, regain the weight they lost from fad diets and such after 5 years.

Diets don't work over the long term. You may see a few weeks or even months of weight loss, but people who go on diets generally end up going back to their old eating habits and gain back the pounds they lost. Diets take the "self" out of self-care behavior. If you give your diet the power in your life, then you are not making choices; they are being made for you *by the diet.* In order to change eating behaviors for life, *you* have to be in the driver's seat, not your diet. If you are not able to control your eating desires, you may regain weight after finishing the diet or sabotage yourself while following it. You need to listen to yourself and understand your desires if you are going to stay on track.

FOOD FOR THOUGHT

If you want to lose weight, it is no mystery that you need to burn more calories than you currently do. It's a simple calories in/calories out issue. Of course, you can't stop eating to lose weight! Food is our fuel. How much fuel are you giving your body? Does your body have the engine of a VW bug that only needs enough gas to drive for 30 minutes, but instead you are filling it up like it's a Hummer heading out on a road trip? To start losing weight (and stop gaining pounds), you'll need to make sure your gas tank only gets the amount of fuel it needs.

So, how do I lose weight?

There are countless ways to lose weight, but great examples can be found in the National Weight Control Registry (www.nwcr.ws), a group that studies people who have lost at least 30 pounds and kept it off for 1 year or longer. There is no single way that they all lost weight and kept it off, but certain things are common among a majority of members. Here's a short list:

- Follow a mostly low-calorie, low-fat diet.
- Eat breakfast every day.
- Weigh yourself at least once a week.
- Watch fewer than 10 hours of TV a week.
- Get an average of 1 hour of exercise per day (usually in the form of walking).

Because you have diabetes, one of the first steps you should take is to find a registered dietitian (RD), who can help you assess your diet and help you create a personalized meal plan. If you don't have an RD already, ask your health care team about how to make this invaluable professional part of your team.

Where am I now?

Do you know how to determine if you are overweight? Body mass index (BMI) is used to measure a person's level of obesity based on his or her height and weight. It is a pretty good way of determining whether a person is overweight. It is calculated by taking weight in kilograms and dividing it by the square of height in meters. But you don't have to do all of that math; instead, you can just look at the following table or find BMI calculators online.

BMI Table

Find your height in feet and inches on the left and then follow along the column until you reach your weight in pounds. The number in the box indicates your BMI.

	140	150	160	170	180	190	200	210	220	230	240	250	260	270	280	290	300
4'6"	34	36	39	41	43	46	48	51	53	56	58	60	63	65	68	70	72
4'8"	31	34	36	38	40	43	45	47	49	52	54	56	58	61	63	65	67
4'10"	29	31	34	36	38	40	42	44	46	48	50	52	54	57	59	61	63
5'	27	29	31	33	35	37	39	41	43	45	47	49	51	53	55	57	59
5'2"	26	27	29	31	33	35	37	38	40	42	44	46	48	49	51	53	55
5'4"	24	26	28	29	31	33	34	36	38	40	41	43	45	46	48	50	52
5'6"	23	24	26	27	29	31	32	34	36	37	39	40	42	44	45	47	49
5'8"	21	23	24	26	27	29	30	32	34	35	37	38	40	41	43	44	46
5'10"	20	22	23	24	26	27	29	30	32	33	35	36	37	39	40	42	43
6'	19	20	22	23	24	26	27	28	30	31	33	34	36	37	38	39	41
6'2"	18	19	21	22	23	24	26	27	28	30	31	32	33	35	36	37	39
6'4"	17	18	20	21	22	23	24	26	27	28	29	30	32	33	34	35	37
6'6"	16	17	19	20	21	22	23	24	25	27	28	29	30	31	32	34	35
6'8"	15	17	18	19	20	21	22	23	24	25	26	28	29	30	31	32	33

BMI categories

Less than 18.4 kg/m^2 = underweight

18.5 to 24.9 kg/m^2 = healthy weight

25 to 29.9 kg/m^2 = overweight

30 to 39.9 kg/m^2 = obese

Over 40 kg/m^2 = extremely obese

Wait. People say that BMI is always wrong.

The BMI was originally developed in the 1840s by the Belgian polymath (a person who has encyclopedic knowledge), Adolphe Quetelet, in his studies of social physics. Since then, it has become widely used. One chart doesn't fit all, but BMI is pretty reliable in people who are overweight and/or physically inactive. For the elderly and the very ill, their bone densities and body frames can make BMI less accurate. Athletes are often considered overweight according to BMI because they have more muscles, which weigh more than fat.

Wouldn't I be better off on a low-carb, high-protein diet?

Not exactly. Low-carb, high-protein diets are effective at helping you lose weight for up to one year, but they also go hand-in-hand with higher fat intake, which people should try to avoid. Not only does fat contain more calories per gram than carbohydrate, but it can also increase insulin resistance and lead to clogged arteries and such.

The other important issue to consider when it comes to low-carb, high-protein diets is that they limit the variety of healthy food choices you take in. You'd miss out on nutrient-dense foods like some vegetables, fruits, and high-fiber starches. Fiber helps lower cholesterol levels and prevents constipation.

THE IMPORTANCE OF MEAL PLANNING

What did you eat in the last 24 hours? Did you make any impulsive decisions about your food choices? Did you skip a meal? Having a plan for your meals is an important key to success. It's like planning for retirement. It takes a little thought, time, and investment, but down the road that meal plan will have saved your life.

A nutritionally balanced meal plan for people with diabetes helps with weight management, which in turn helps people manage their diabetes! There is reason for this. Excess weight makes it more difficult for the body to use its limited supply of available insulin. If you are overweight, losing 7% of your weight (in many cases, just 10–15 pounds) will be the ticket to lowering blood glucose levels. Many studies show this can be accomplished by getting at least 30 minutes of exercise (this includes walking) a day.

If you learn to love your body, many positive things will follow. You can turn things around one meal, one workout, and one food choice at a time. You've got built-in safety devices: your head, arms, and legs. Your head tells you what it wants to eat. Your legs have to take you to the food. Your arms bring the food to your mouth. Make *health-conscious* choices. As you move forward, avoid letting yesterday's mistakes put up road blocks to your health today. If you made some unhealthy choices the day before (or even the meal before), don't beat yourself up over it. Simply move on to the next chance you get to make a healthy choice.

PERSONAL GOAL

This week (date _____), I decided I can (*check one*):

☐ Integrate healthy food choices into my lifestyle.
☐ Wait 15 minutes before treating myself to unhealthy snacks (even a five-minute distraction can thwart a craving). If I can't wait, I'll have just a few bites and savor them.
☐ Brush my teeth after eating to send a message to my brain that the meal is over.
☐ Call a registered dietitian (RD) to help me get a weight management and meal plan.
☐ Plan at least three days' worth of meals ahead of time this week.
☐ Start a food and activity diary to track what I eat and what activities I do.
☐ Avoid skipping breakfast and eat most of my calories before 7 p.m.
☐ Other: _____.

 The grocery store gets in the way of my meal planning.

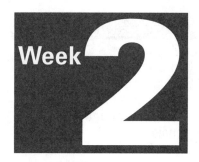

Week 2

The Cost of Junk Food

 Want to think twice about unhealthy food choices? Just try thinking about how much activity it will take to "cover" the calories that you get from junk food.

Americans get 30% of their calories from junk food (nutrient-poor foods that are high in fat, sugar, or both). Only 10% of caloric intake comes from fruit and vegetables. That's terrible! A third of our calories are empty—devoid of vitamins and minerals. We need to turn this problem around, so that junk food constitutes a much smaller portion of our daily intake.

This list, based on a 160-pound adult, estimates how much activity it would take to burn the calories from these goodies. If you weigh less, you burn fewer calories, and if you weigh more, you burn more calories. So, next time you're glancing at a candy bar or a bag of chips, don't just think about how much money that package will cost you, but also about how much physical activity it'll cost.

100 Calories IN	=	100 Calories OUT

• 4 Hershey's kisses
• 2 mini Reese's peanut butter cups
• 3 pieces of Bazooka gum
• 1 small package of peanut M&Ms (0.7 oz)
• Glass of wine (red or white)
• 1 Corona Light beer
• 1 Sierra Nevada Pale Ale beer
• 4 oz margarita
		• 2,000 steps
		• 8 minutes of jogging
		• 10 minutes of
		  o basketball
		  o chopping wood
		  o dancing (aerobic)
		  o swimming at a moderate pace
		• 20 minutes of walking or weightlifting
		• 1 hour of bowling

200 Calories IN = 200 Calories OUT	

• 1 medium, plain croissant
• 4 Oreo cookies
• 18 Pringle's potato chips
• 1 KFC biscuit
• 1 slice of cheese or chicken pizza
• 1.8 oz bag of Skittles
• 1 Pete's Wicked Ale beer
	• 4,000 steps
	• 16 minutes of jogging
	• 26 minutes of
	  ○ skating (ice or rollerblade)
	  ○ skiing (water or downhill)
	  ○ tennis
	  ○ shoveling snow
	  ○ biking (about 10 mph)
	• 30 minutes of
	  ○ gardening
	  ○ golfing (pull/carry clubs)
	  ○ hiking
	• 40 minutes of walking or weightlifting
	• 70 minutes of
	  ○ golfing (power cart)

300 Calories IN = 300 Calories OUT	

• 1 Snicker's candy bar (2.07 oz)
• 1 old-fashioned cake donut
• 1 almond-filled croissant
• 5 Pepperidge Farm Milano cookies
• 1 McDonald's apple bran muffin (4 oz)
• 1/2 cup Haagen-Dazs ice cream
	• 6,000 steps
	• 24 minutes of jogging
	• 30 minutes of
	  ○ swimming
	  ○ basketball
	• 39 minutes of
	  ○ skating (ice or rollerblade)
	  ○ skiing (water or downhill)
	  ○ tennis
	  ○ shoveling snow
	  ○ biking (about 10 mph)
	• 45 minutes of gardening
	• 60 minutes of walking or weightlifting
	• 3 hours of bowling

400 Calories IN = 400 Calories OUT	
• 1 Kit Kat bar (2.8 oz) • 1 Nestle's brownie (3.5 oz) • 1 piece of tiramisu (5 oz) • 1 Starbuck's Green Tea Frappuccino (16 oz)	• 8,000 steps • 32 minutes of jogging • 56 minutes of biking • 64 minutes golfing (pull/carry clubs) or hiking • 1 hour, 50 minutes of social dancing • 2 hours, 20 minutes of golfing (power cart)

Warning! This exercise is meant to clarify how quickly those calories from junk foods build up. Its purpose is to keep in mind how much specific foods affect your balance of calories in versus calories out. Its purpose is not to let you justify eating as much junk food as you want and then promising yourself that you'll "cancel it out" with exercise.

I love my junk food. Are there any healthier options?

Here's a list of the top five junk foods and alternative choices.

Junk	Healthier Options	Why
Regular soda	Diet soda, water, sugar-free beverages, carbonated water, tea	Unless you are hypoglycemic, your body doesn't need the 8 tsp of sugar contained in a 12-oz soda. Drinking water helps hydrate the body and keeps the kidneys happy.
Sweets, desserts, and pastries	Go with fruit instead or low-fat or nonfat yogurt. Switch to dark chocolate in small amounts.	Fruit has no fat, few calories, and lots of fiber. Sweets are loaded with fat, sugar, and calories, which is the opposite of what you need. Dark chocolate has antioxidants and may benefit the blood vessels.
Fast food (hamburgers and fries)	Ask for your burger without cheese or mayonnaise. Try veggie burgers. Ask for a salad with low-fat dressing. Share the fries.	You can avoid lots of hidden calories, carbohydrates, and fat. And salt. And guilt. Get a fast food nutrition guide or ask for a nutrition guide at your favorite fast food places so you can identify healthier choices.
Pizza	Go for lower-fat (vegetables) and fewer toppings. Share the pizza and avoid eating the whole thing in one sitting.	Pizza is the gift that keeps on giving. Pizza can raise blood glucose levels for hours and contains lots of fat and cholesterol.
Potato chips	Baked potato chips or a baked potato (*not loaded* with toppings)	Potato chips offer next to nothing in nutrients, except for fat, fat, and fat, plus some oil and salt. Baked potatoes are a healthy choice when topped only with veggies, baked beans, or cottage cheese.

PERSONAL GOAL

This week (date _____), I decided I can (*check one*):

☐ Burn about 200 calories by walking to work or by walking during my break at work.
☐ Clear my cupboards of junk food and fill them with healthier options.
☐ Eat fast food only once a week.
☐ Order a calorie, fat gram, and carbohydrate counting book.
☐ Try an exercise I once enjoyed but haven't done in a while.
☐ Other: _____.

Sex burns 4 calories a minute. It's going to take some work to burn 200 calories a day.

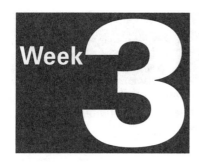

Week 3

Cholesterol Medications

Cholesterol building up in your blood vessels is like a smoldering fire. If ignored, it can overcome you when you least expect it. You can help put out the fire of high cholesterol (fat swimming in your blood) with one of these common cholesterol medications:

Types of cholesterol medicines	Brand name (generic name)	Possible side effects or issues
Statins (work by reducing the liver's ability to make LDL cholesterol)	**Crestor** (rosuvastatin) **Lipitor** (atorvastatin) **Lescol** (fluvastatin) **Mevacor** (lovastatin) **Pravachol** (pravastatin) **Zocor** (simvastatin)	If you have muscle pain, notify your health care provider immediately. Use caution when combined with fibric acid derivatives, bile acid sequestrants, or erythromycin because of a rare and potentially fatal condition called rhabdomyolysis. Usually taken at bedtime. Side effects can include insomnia, fatigue, depression, rash, and headaches.
Cholesterol Absorption Inhibitors (reduce total and LDL cholesterol levels by limiting absorption of cholesterol from food)	**Zetia** (ezetimibe)	Can be used alone or in combination with other drugs.

Types of cholesterol medicines	Brand name (generic name)	Possible side effects or issues
Fibric Acid Derivatives (reduce triglycerides and raise HDL cholesterol, but have little effect on LDL cholesterol)	**Lopid** (gemfibrozil) **Tricor** (fenofibrate)	If you have muscle pain, notify your health care provider immediately.
Bile Acid Sequestrants (lower LDL cholesterol by binding to bile in the small intestine and preventing it from being absorbed into circulation)	**LoCholest** (cholestra-mine) **Questran** (cholestra-mine) **Prevalite** (cholestra-mine) **Welchol** (colesevelam)	May cause constipation and stomach upset. Taken once or twice a day with meals. Welchol may reduce blood glucose levels by 18 mg/dl after eating.
Nicotinic Acid (also known as niacin, increases HDL cholesterol levels, lowers LDL cholesterol, and lowers triglycerides)	**Niaspan and others** (nicotinic acid)	May increase insulin resistance and increase blood glucose levels. Frequent side effects include facial flushing and other skin conditions and worsening of gout or peptic ulcers. Take with food.
Combination	**Advicor** (lovastatin/ niacin) **Vytorin** (ezetimibe/ simvastatin)	See descriptions above.

PERSONAL GOAL

This week (date _____), I decided I can (*check one*):

☐ Call my health care provider immediately if I am on one of these drugs and have muscle pain.

☐ Tell my health care provider, certified diabetes educator, or pharmacist about any possible side effects I might be having.

☐ Get copies of my recent liver function test and make sure I have one taken at least once a year.

☐ Take statins at bedtime.

☐ Take bile acid sequestrants with food.

☐ Report a flushed face, upset stomach, or constipation to my doctor.

☐ Ask my doctor or health care provider about the next step in controlling cholesterol.

☐ Refill my cholesterol drug prescriptions before they run out.

☐ Other: _____.

☺ **Mom gave me blue eyes, hammer toes, and high cholesterol. Dad gave me his love of fried foods. I've got a long road to travel.**

Eye of the Beholder

How can my doctor check my visual ability?

Three main types of examinations are used to determine eye health.

1. Visual acuity test. This is the fancy name for that eye chart that you read from a distance with different rows of letters and numbers. It checks if you have 20/20 vision.

2. *Dilated eye exam.* Eyedrops are used to widen your pupils so that the doctor can check your retina and optic nerve for damage by using a special magnifying lens. Your vision may be blurred and you may experience a headache after the exam.

3. *Tonometry.* This test measures eye pressure and can indicate whether you have glaucoma or other pressure-related problems.

What are some common eye problems related to diabetes?

- *Blurry vision.* High blood glucose levels may cause blurry vision. Blurry vision can go away after blood glucose levels return to the target range, providing they haven't been high for years.
- *Cataracts.* A clouding of the lens is twice as likely to happen in people with diabetes and at a younger age than in those without diabetes. Cataracts can be surgically removed.
- *Glaucoma.* A condition in which increased pressure in the eye damages the optic nerve (the main nerve in the eye) over a long time. The first symptom of glaucoma is reduced vision out of the corners of the eyes. Glaucoma can be treated with medications or surgery. If left untreated, glaucoma can lead to blindness.
- *Retinopathy.* The most common eye problem associated with diabetes is retinopathy, in which the tiny blood vessels leak fluid into the light-sensing lining in the back of the eye (called the retina). This can lead to vision loss. In the early stage, it's called background retinopathy and typically no symptoms are present. In the advanced stage, proliferative retinopathy can develop, in which the eye grows new blood vessels that are fragile, tend to grow in the wrong places, and bleed into the eyeball. If left untreated, this can lead to blindness. With timely treatment, blindness can often be prevented.

What signs should I watch for?

Often, there are no early signs of vision problems. Report any of these to your doctor:

- Blurred or double vision
- Pain or pressure in the eyes

- Flashing lights or rings of light in the vision
- Difficulty seeing things out of the corner of the eyes

What are the treatments for retinopathy?

Laser surgery is a common and effective way to deal with retinopathy. You can protect your sight by having yearly checkups with an ophthalmologist.

PERSONAL GOAL

This week (date _____), I decided I can (*check one*):

☐ Check my blood glucose if my vision suddenly becomes blurry.

☐ Tell my eye doctor if I don't see well out of the corners of my eyes, have double or blurry vision, have eye pain or pressure, or see flashing lights.

☐ Call my ophthalmologist to make my yearly appointment for a dilated eye exam.

☐ Find an ophthalmologist by calling Eye Care America at 1-800-222-3937.

☐ Reduce my fat intake, which will lower my cholesterol and help me keep my eyes healthy.

☐ Keep my eyes lubricated—if they are dry—with a normal saline-type solution (not brands that advertise reducing redness).

☐ If I'm pregnant and in my first or third trimester, I'll get an eye exam.

☐ Other: _____.

I can see clearly now, the cholesterol is gone.

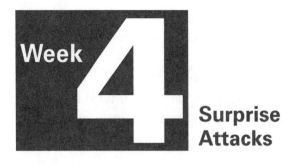

Week **4**

Surprise Attacks

What's the connection between diabetes and cardiovascular disease?

People are often shocked to learn that between 66% and 75% of people with diabetes die from cardiovascular complications, such as heart attacks and strokes. Insulin resistance is the main issue with type 2 diabetes and is associated with atherosclerosis (the technical name for arteries that are clogged by fatty deposits). When arteries are narrowed, less oxygen can be delivered to the heart and brain. Plaques can then dislodge or create an environment in which blood flow is completely blocked, leading to a heart attack or stroke.

What is a heart attack?

A heart attack occurs when part of the heart muscle dies from lack of oxygen. More than one million people in the U.S. have a heart attack (also called a myocardial infarction or MI) every year. It's common to experience angina (temporary chest pain) before having a heart attack, so it's important to listen to your body's signals. Treatment is aimed at increasing circulation and oxygen back to the heart, thinning blood to prevent clotting, reducing the workload of the heart, and managing blood pressure and cholesterol.

What is a stroke?

A stroke (or cerebral vascular accident or CVA) occurs when the blood flow to an area in the brain stops, either because an artery bursts or is blocked. The number of stroke victims has decreased over the past 45 years thanks to widespread use of medications for high blood pressure and high cholesterol. Women have a higher risk of strokes (1 in 5 women have a stroke) than men (1 in 10).

Depending on the area of the brain that does not get life-sustaining oxygen, the level of destruction can vary from loss of speech and vision to paralysis of a single arm or leg. In the worst cases, strokes result in coma and death. Symptoms include a sudden change in vision, a severe headache, sudden numbness on one side of the body, difficulty understanding what someone just told you, trouble with balance and coordination, and difficulty speaking.

People who have suffered a heart attack have a 44% risk for having a stroke within the next 30 days. New technology and treatments are available to help minimize the devastating impact of a stroke. The best treatment is to never have a stroke, so we should focus on prevention. If you or someone you know has had a stroke, there's a high risk of having another, so following measures to control diabetes, blood pressure, and cholesterol is more important than ever.

How do I prevent heart attacks and strokes?

Besides following a nutritious diet, being active most days, and maintaining target A1C levels, these steps can further protect your heart and brain:

- Take one baby aspirin tablet (81 or 162 mg) every day if your health care provider approves it.
- Reduce stress.
- Avoid smoking and secondhand smoke.
- Eat fish three times a week or an ounce of walnuts a day to get your dose of protective omega-3s up.
- Improve your cholesterol. Reduce LDL cholesterol by 10% and your risk of heart-related events will go down by 25%. For every 1 milligram increase in HDL cholesterol, the risk for cardiovascular disease drops by 2–3%.
- Have a sleep study done to check for sleep apnea (which is linked to sudden cardiac death and stroke).
- Brush and floss your teeth.
- Know your blood pressure.

Have a heart and don't tell me what can go wrong.

Your Virtual Community

With the click of a button, you can find tons of information about diabetes on the Internet and on select television channels. Being informed about diabetes can help you take care of yourself, but it's always important to be objective and careful when you research. Not all of those sources out there are reliable or can be trusted. Consider the source of the information when you are researching. Does it come from a respected organization or does the information come from an individual who is an expert in living with the disease? These are things to keep in mind as you surf the Internet.

Be careful when reading about cures and treatments for diabetes on the Internet. Some companies are more concerned about making a profit than curing or helping people with diabetes. The same goes for miracle dietary supplements and products with claims that they can cure or prevent diabetes. In general, that old mail fraud rule applies: if it sounds too good to be true, then it probably is.

Great resources for people with diabetes

American Diabetes Association (ADA)
www.diabetes.org
1-800-232-3472
This site describes new developments in diabetes, including current research, and offers access to the ADA's information center and links to state affiliates. It lists the organization's consumer and professional publications, with articles from the current issue of *Diabetes Forecast* as well as some from past issues. If you want the official, science-backed standard of care, start your engine search here!

American Association of Diabetes Educators
www.diabeteseducator.org
1-800-338-3633
The professional association dedicated to ensuring the delivery of high-quality diabetes education. You can find the nearest certified diabetes educator by clicking on the "Find a Diabetes Educator" link under the About Diabetes Education tab at the top of the page.

American Dietetic Association
www.eatright.org
1-800-877-1600
Provides you with a link to nutrition and health. Check out the Food and Nutrition tab and tap into the wealth of consumer resources.

Diabetes Exercise & Sports Association
www.diabetes-exercise.org
1-800-898-4322
Information provided by this organization focuses on diabetes and the role of exercise in enhancing health.

Diabetes Health Magazine
www.DiabetesHealth.com
1-800-488-8468 (customer service)
A monthly magazine that focuses on living well with diabetes, *Diabetes Health* includes information, resources, and products. Various articles from current issues and an article archive are available.

Diabetes Health Monitor
http://www.healthmonitor.com/diabetes
A comprehensive website with a free magazine that is distributed six times a year.

dLife
www.dlife.com
This site offers inspiration, opportunity to ask an expert, valuable offers, and more for people with diabetes. You can look up any food item or watch cooking demonstrations. It is the only cable diabetes program available. Check your local listings and tune in on Sundays on CNBC.

Joslin Diabetes Center
www.joslin.org
This center in Boston is an internationally known institution devoted to the study and treatment of diabetes. It provides contact information for Joslin satellite sites and affiliate centers, lists research studies needing volunteers, and offers discussion groups moderated by a diabetes educator and social worker. A special feature is a "Beginner's Guide" for those newly diagnosed.

Juvenile Diabetes Research Foundation International (JDRF)
www.jdrf.org
1-800-533-2873
The JDRF website offers specific information about diabetes in children as well as information about the not-for-profit voluntary agency's activities, research, advocacy, and publications.

MedicAlert

www.medicalert.org

1-888-633-4298

This is a not-for-profit organization whose mission is to provide services to protect and save lives. Members provide critical health information that, in an emergency situation, can be released to providers 24 hours a day anywhere in the world. Also includes an online system for ordering customized emblems (bracelets and necklaces) for the purpose of identifying the specific medical conditions and/or allergies of the wearer.

My Pyramid

www.mypyramid.gov

Take a step inside the new food pyramid to help you choose the foods and servings that are right for you. Helps you get the most nutrition for your calories.

National Diabetes Information Clearinghouse

www.diabetes.niddk.nih.gov

1-800-860-8747

An information service of the National Institute of Diabetes and Digestive and Kidney Diseases, part of the National Institutes of Health, the Clearinghouse provides information about diabetes, care, treatment, and medical resources. It includes an online system for ordering publications.

Medlineplus.com

www.nlm.nih.gov/medlineplus/diabetes.html

This National Institutes of Health website provides current and understandable medical information for people with diabetes and their families, including an online slide show tutorial. It also offers a drug database, links to a medical encyclopedia and dictionary, and resource directories.

PERSONAL GOAL

This week (date _____), I decided I can (*check one*):

☐ Subscribe to a free or paid diabetes journal as a way to stay current with the latest in diabetes research, treatment, and technology.

☐ Call any diabetes journal and ask if they have a free issue for me to preview.

☐ Ask my certified diabetes educator for a free diabetes magazine.

☐ Ask my local library or hospital for a video or DVD about diabetes.

☐ Join a virtual diabetes support group moderated by a diabetes educator.

☐ Watch an online video about diabetes.

☐ Ask my pharmacist for a diabetes magazine.

☐ Other: _____.

Waves or the web...I'm still afraid of the sharks.

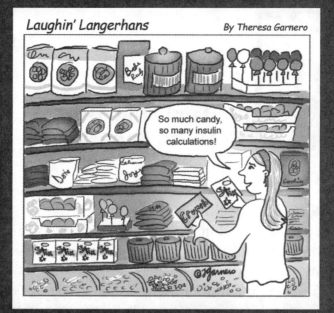

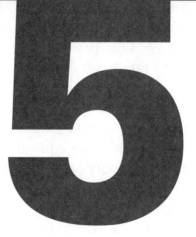

Month **5**

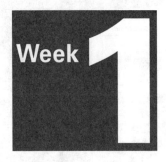

Week 1

Protein: From Beef to Beans to Barracuda

What is protein?

Protein is found in the meat and beans food group and contains materials needed to build up, maintain, and replace the body's cells. Cells are the smallest component of our bodies and the fundamental unit of living tissue, visible only under a microscope. Protein is necessary for the formation of hormones, enzymes, antibodies, muscles, skin, hair, nails, and internal organs.

How much protein do I need?

The Recommended Dietary Allowance from protein is about 46 grams per day, although more or less may be needed based on age, sex, and physical activity. Adults should get about 10–35% of their calories from protein.

It's pretty difficult to break down everything you eat into a percentage of calories, so take the easy way out: follow the Plate Method (from Day 15) or try using the ounce equivalents as advised by the new food pyramid at MyPyramid.gov. Here's how it works:

Count 1-ounce equivalents of protein to add up to the recommended 5 ounce equivalents for women or 6 ounce equivalents for men per day. Men are allowed more protein so they'll have extra energy to take out the trash. Not really. It has to do with men having more muscle mass. Be sure to choose lean protein sources when adding up your 5- or 6-ounce equivalents.

Ounce-Protein Equivalent Examples	Meat	Poultry	Fish	Egg/Nuts	Beans/Tofu
1	1 ounce lean beef	1 ounce skinless turkey or chicken	1 ounce cooked fish or shellfish	1 egg; 1 Tbsp peanut butter; 12 almonds; 24 pistachios; 7 walnut halves; 2 Tbsp pumpkin or sunflower seeds	1/2 cup cooked beans (refried, black, white, pinto, kidney) or peas (lentils, split peas, chickpeas); 1/2 cup tofu; 1/3 cup hummus
2	2 ounces cooked pork or ham	2 ounces skinless turkey or chicken	1/2 can of drained tuna	4 Tbsp (1/8 cup) pumpkin or sunflower seeds	1 soy or tofu burger
3	1 small hamburger	1 small chicken breast	1 small trout		1/4 cup wheat gluten
4	1 small steak (eye of round, filet)	1/2 Cornish game hen	1 salmon steak		

So, if you're a woman, you can have 4 Tbsp of sunflower seeds and a small chicken breast to meet your protein requirements for the day. A man can have 4 Tbsp of sunflower seeds and a small steak instead. Other combinations are possible, and this isn't even a complete list!

Does that look like too little food? Remember that we also get protein in our diets from other sources, including dairy products, starches, and some vegetables. These 5–6 ounces are based on the assumption that people will get extra protein from these other sources. In the U.S., we have no trouble getting enough protein: we consume almost twice the amount of protein—and fat for that matter—than is needed. Protein doesn't raise blood glucose like carbohydrates, but you need to be on the lookout for fat. Each gram of protein and carbohydrate contain 4 calories, but fat contains 9 calories per gram. Those calories can add up quickly.

What is considered a lean source of protein?

Get yourself lean and mean by choosing protein sources that are baked, broiled, barbequed (while holding off on the BBQ sauce), steamed, or grilled. For all meats, trim off excess fat and remove skin from poultry. For the following selections, try to avoid fried dishes:

- Beef round
- Fresh pork or ham
- Sirloin
- Skinless chicken or turkey breast
- Tofu or wheat gluten

What about fish?

The omega-3 fat content of fish has been shown to help protect against coronary artery disease. Generally, the darker the meat on a fish (like salmon, herring, and mackerel), the more omega-3 fatty acids it has. Conversely, the lighter the meat (such as cod and flounder), the less omega-3 it'll have. Some fish, like trout and salmon, contain more fat than some beef choices. So if you do eat fish, consider making healthy choices. Fried calamari may taste yummy, but can your arteries afford that luxury?

AN ARGUMENT FOR A VEGETARIAN DIET

Vegetarians are herbivores. They do not eat animal flesh. Ovo-lacto vegetarians include dairy products, such as eggs, cheese, and milk, in their diets, whereas vegans do not eat (and often don't wear or use) anything of animal origin. Research suggests that vegetarianism makes for good health. The cornerstone of a vegetarian diet is vegetables.

Those who eat meat have *three* times the obesity rate of vegetarians and *nine* times the obesity rate of vegans. Vegetarians have the lowest rate of coronary artery disease of any group, with a fraction of the heart attack rate and 40% less cancer than those who eat meat. Plus, on average, vegetarians and vegans live 6–10 years longer than meat eaters. The downside? The longer you live, the more taxes you'll pay.

Many people are concerned that following a vegetarian diet means that it will be tough to get enough protein or calcium. This is true for people who do not carefully put together their meal plans, but vitamin and mineral supplements can be used to ensure that you get the proper nutrients. In general, though, following a healthy vegetarian diet will provide enough protein and calcium, which can be found in tofu products, whole-wheat bread, oatmeal, beans, legumes, nuts, and broccoli. If you eat a variety of unrefined grains, legumes, seeds, nuts, and vegetables throughout the day, even if one food is low in a particular essential nutrient, another food will make up this deficit. There are tons of vegetarian options out there, including tofu, wheat gluten, tempeh, Quorn, textured vegetable protein, egg replacers, and nondairy "dairy" products. Try a few; you may be surprised by how much you like them.

PERSONAL GOAL

This week (date _____), I decided I can (*check one*):

☐ Reduce my protein intake.
☐ Try something different just once; twice if I like it.
☐ Support those soybean farmers: try tofu!
☐ Visit www.MyPyramid.gov for an inside look at the food pyramid.
☐ Try a wheat gluten dish.
☐ Eat leaner cuts of meat.
☐ Experiment with other protein sources.
☐ Try an egg substitute.
☐ Remove the skin from poultry.
☐ Other: _____.

Albert Einstein was a vegetarian who found the relativity of wheat gluten as a hair product.

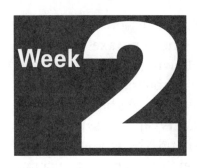

Week **2**

Exercise Fundamentals

When is the best time to exercise?

The best time for exercise is when you're most likely to get that exercise done. Many people prefer to get their exercise done first thing in the morning, so the rest of their day doesn't interfere with their exercise routine. Another popular option is to exercise after work. Try to pick a time that fits your schedule and works for you.

Do I need a pre-exercise snack?

Some people do require a pre-exercise snack. It depends on your blood glucose level at the time, the planned physical activity, when you had your last meal, and the intensity of the workout. Consider having a pre-exercise snack to prevent hypoglycemia if any of the follow conditions applies to you:

- Your glucose is less than 100 mg/dl.
- You will exercise before a meal.
- You will be active for more than 30 minutes (especially if more than an hour).
- Your medication or insulin is peaking.

Based on a 150-pound person, you'd need about 30–40 grams of carbohydrate snack for one hour of activity. If you plan on 30 minutes, you'd need 15–20 grams of carbohydrate. The best way to know if your snack is enough is to check your blood glucose before and after exercise. If the glucose levels are similar, it's the right amount of snack. If your blood glucose level is too low, you need more carbohydrate, and if it's too high, you need less carbohydrate.

Warm up your engine.

Warming up prepares your body for increased activity by bringing oxygen into your muscles. It reduces risk for injury. Do five minutes of warm-up activities, such as knee lifts, arm windmills, trunk rotations, jumping jacks, or walking or slowly jogging in place.

Stretch it.

After a brief warm-up, another five minutes of stretching makes the exercise more comfortable. Stretch slowly, and don't bounce or hold your breath. Go from head-to-toe with gentle movements to stretch your neck, shoulders, back, legs, ankles, and feet. An excellent resource for healthy workouts is the Training Fan (www.trainingfan.com), which includes 20 stretches, 84 exercises, 3 complete preset workouts, and training logs to track your progress.

How long should I exercise?

If you haven't been getting much physical activity recently, you'll need to start slowly and with realistic goals. It's not practical to jump from not exercising to 60 minutes a day. Give yourself time to build up. Start with five minutes a day. After a week of that, go up to 10 minutes a day. Continue ramping up until you're getting at least 30 minutes a day.

For the best health benefits, strive for 30 minutes of moderate activity a day, such as walking briskly, golfing (carry or pull the clubs), hiking, gardening, bicycling, weight training, and light aerobic workouts. To maintain a healthy weight, you should be looking at 60 minutes a day, and if you want to lose weight, at least 90 minutes a day is suggested.

Cool off!

Cool down after exercising by doing five minutes of slow walking or stretches.

Stay hydrated.

When you exercise, your body needs more fluid to keep it cool. Drink water before and after exercise to prevent dehydration. It helps to drink fluids during exercise as well.

What exercise factors can affect my glucose?

- The less fit you are, the greater the impact exercise will have on your blood glucose levels. This means as you get in shape, your exercise-related blood glucose fluctuations should decrease.
- If you only do one type of exercise, you will see an increased effect on your blood glucose levels if you try a different type of exercise. If you jog routinely and then start swimming, the swimming will have a bigger effect on blood glucose levels.
- Your pre-exercise blood glucose level has an enormous impact on your post-exercise levels. Know where you start!
- Drinking alcohol the previous day can affect blood glucose levels.
- Exercising the previous day can have a lasting effect.
- Your hydration state (the caffeine in a triple cappuccino can dehydrate you for an afternoon workout and increase blood glucose levels).

Exercise improves insulin sensitivity (whether it's your own or the insulin you inject), heart function, muscle mass, and weight management. What are you willing to change to make that happen?

PERSONAL GOAL

This week (date _____), I decided I can
(*check one*):

- ☐ Check my blood glucose level if I feel nervous, shaky, or hungry during my workout or several hours after and treat for lows if it's less than 70 mg/dl.
- ☐ Check my blood glucose level, have a 15- to 20-gram carbohydrate snack before activity, and recheck my blood glucose level afterward. I will adjust my snack size until my before and after blood glucose levels are similar.
- ☐ Drink a glass of water 30 minutes before and after I exercise.
- ☐ Schedule an appointment to exercise when I'm least likely to cancel it.
- ☐ Squeeze in a 10-minute break for a brisk walk.
- ☐ Warm up for five minutes by doing gentle jumping jacks.
- ☐ Stretch before my shower every day over the next week.
- ☐ Sign up for a dance class.

The note I made to myself is illegible.

Week 3

Alternate Site Testing

 Want to give your fingers a rest from being pricked for all of that blood glucose monitoring? You may want to think about alternate site testing.

Why bother?

Your fingertips have more nerve endings than the forearm. For some people, their work is not conducive to fingersticks (for example, musicians, computer techs, health care workers, environmental engineers). Also, many people feel that alternative site testing hurts less than the traditional side-of-the-finger route.

The amount of blood required to perform an alternate site test is minimal. However, due to decreased circulation in the arm, you may need to rub your arm before using the lancet device to get an adequate blood sample and obtain accurate results.

How do I know if I should use alternate site testing?

Try it once to see if you like it. Some people love it; others report that it takes a little more time to get used to, can leave a small bruise, or increases tenderness in the testing area. You won't know until you give it a try. Here are other factors that can determine whether alternate site testing is the right path for you:

- Your body hair. If you have too much, you may smear the drop of blood and make it nearly impossible to get a clear reading.
- Access to alternative sites. Do you wear long sleeves or bulky sweaters that could make it difficult to get to your arm?
- You bruise or bleed easily. A pinprick may turn into a bloody mess that is difficult to cover with a bandage.

Can I use alternate site testing all the time?

Under certain circumstances, alternate site testing is not recommended, especially during rapid fluctuations in blood glucose. The arm responds to glucose levels more slowly than the fingertip. You might feel low and test your arm, but the low reading hasn't made it to your arm yet.

Do not use alternate site testing if:

- You have a history of hypoglycemia unawareness (you don't know when you are low).
- You think your blood glucose is low.
- Your result doesn't match how you feel (try confirming the number with a fingerstick measurement).
- You are testing after exercise (you won't get an accurate reading from an alternate site).

When in doubt, always test on the fingertip.

PERSONAL GOAL

This week (date _____), I decided I can (*check one*):

- ☐ Find out if my meter has an alternate site testing option.
- ☐ Make sure I have the right equipment for alternate site testing (sometimes a different lancet device or attachment is required).
- ☐ Rub the alternate site to increase circulation before checking my blood glucose levels.
- ☐ Learn how to do the alternate site test.
- ☐ Avoid alternate site testing if I feel low, if I just finished exercising, or if I don't feel well.
- ☐ Give my fingers a break today.
- ☐ Other: _____.

Use someone else for your alternate site test.

Insulin Is In

 At least 30% of people with type 2 diabetes need insulin. The hormone insulin is life sustaining—we need it like we need air. If your body is not making enough insulin, you have to get it somehow. Insulin is the most powerful tool out there for managing diabetes.

One of the most common hurdles to starting insulin therapy is the fear of needles. This is understandable, but technology has vastly improved methods of insulin delivery with much smaller, shorter needles and needle-less systems. Finding a "comfortable needle" is no longer an oxymoron. So, before you completely write off insulin therapy, think about the powerful control it'll bring to your diabetes self-care. There are a lot of myths surrounding insulin, but don't let them stop you from getting the help you need. Insulin doesn't cause complications; having long periods of high blood glucose levels does. A certified diabetes educator or a member of your health care team can help you learn how to take insulin.

If I need insulin, does that mean my diabetes is really bad?

No. It just means that your pancreas is not producing as much insulin anymore, and injecting insulin will help you in your diabetes self-care. You didn't do anything wrong.

What are the types of insulin?

Insulin falls into two broad categories:

- *Short-acting (mealtime or correction) insulin*—covers your meals or corrects a high blood glucose reading.
- *Long-acting (background or basal) insulin*—provides a steady level of insulin throughout the day and/or night.

How much insulin do I need?

Based on your glucose patterns, your health care provider will decide the type of insulin approach to take. If most or all of your blood glucose levels are above target (more than 130 mg/dl before a meal or more than 180 mg/dl two hours after a meal), long-acting insulin

What about Weight Gain and Insulin?

When blood glucose levels are constantly high, the body burns fat for energy. Once a person starts taking insulin, the body is able to get its energy from food rather than fat, so a few pounds return that shouldn't have been lost in the first place. Saying insulin causes weight gain is like saying recovering from the flu causes weight gain.

Once people discover that the flexibility of insulin can cover meal choices—or dessert—they may begin eating extra calories and covering it with insulin. So, if someone does start to gain a little weight in this situation, what caused the weight gain? Certainly not the insulin! It's those little extras in the diet. Insulin also comes with responsibility, just like following a healthy eating plan.

Another possible reason for weight gain associated with insulin therapy is the issue of treating and overtreating hypoglycemia (which can occur when insulin is first prescribed). The calories from glucose tablets and snacks used to treat and prevent lows can cause weight gain. If you are having more than two episodes of hypoglycemia in a week or you have to eat to prevent lows, talk to your health care provider about adjusting your insulin.

is usually prescribed. If you run high after a meal, short-acting insulin is selected. It's common to use both types, because their actions can be combined to bring blood glucose to nearly normal levels.

What is insulin action?

Think of insulin action like popping popcorn. The kernels of corn don't pop all at once. A few kernels pop first, then most pop at once, and a few leftover kernels pop at the end. Similarly, insulin doesn't all work at once. There is a delay; then it starts to kick in (known as *onset*), most of it works at its strongest for a certain amount of time (known as the *peak*), and some of it lingers in your system, but does not have as strong an effect (known as the *duration*).

Insulin type	Brand name (generic name)	Onset	Peak	Duration	Notes
Mealtime or correction Rapid-acting	**Apidra** (glulisine) **Humalog** (lispro) **NovoLog** (aspart)	5–10 minutes	1–2 hours	3–4 hours	If using with a meal, make sure you do not delay the meal. If you are eating out, don't inject until your meal has been delivered. If you skip a meal, skip this, too.
Short-acting	**Humulin** or **Novolin** (regular)	30 minutes	2–4 hours	4–8 hours	
Background or basal Intermediate-acting	**Novolin N** (NPH)	2–4 hours	6–10 hours	Up to 20 hours	Be sure to roll (do not shake) the vial or pen to mix the solution before injecting.
Long-acting	**Lantus** (glargine) **Levemir** (detemir)	1–2 hours	Peak-less	Up to 24 hours	Avoid mixing with other insulins in the same syringe. Take about the same time daily. Don't skip doses.
Combo 70/30 75/25	70% NPH 30% regular 75% NPH 25% lispro	30 minutes	2–12 hours	Up to 24 hours	Roll the vial or pen before use.

Let's stay cool: insulin storage

Bottles (vials). Keep unopened vials of insulin in the refrigerator (36–46°F) and opened ones at room temperature (59–86°F; for glulisine: less than 77°F). Insulin is easier to inject (i.e., less burning sensation) when it is at room temperature. Once a vial has been opened (whether or not it is in the fridge), it is only good for 28 days (except detemir, which can be kept at room temperature for 42 days). This means you need to throw away unused insulin if the expiration date has passed.

If You Need It: U-500

Some people are highly resistant to insulin and require more than 200 units a day. If this applies to you, then regular U-500 insulin (which has five times the strength of the standard U-100 insulin concentration) may be prescribed. U-500 absorbs more slowly, peaks in 5–7 hours, and may last as long as 24 hours. It's usually taken in one to three injections using a different type of syringe that has volume, instead of unit, markings (called a tuberculin syringe). Pre-dinner doses are usually smaller than pre-breakfast doses to minimize the risk of nighttime hypoglycemia. If you need U-500, you need to see a diabetes nurse educator.

Pens. Keep insulin pens at room temperature. Expiration dates vary among different pen manufacturers, so check the package inserts or ask your pharmacist. Generally, 75/25 insulin expires 10 days after opening; 70/30 expires in 14 days; glulisine, lispro, aspart, and regular expire in 28 days; and detemir expires in 42 days.

Where can I inject the insulin?

Insulin should be injected into the abdomen (stomach area), upper or outer arms, outer thighs, and buttocks. Don't inject near scars and stay at least two inches away from your belly button. Rotate your injection sites to avoid developing scar tissue. Pick a general area to use for a month, and then move to another site for another month.

What sites absorb insulin the quickest?

Insulin is absorbed the fastest from the following sites in the following order (from fastest to slowest): abdomen, arms, legs, and buttocks. If you tend to have lower blood glucose levels, you might consider injecting into a site that absorbs more slowly, like the buttocks or thigh. Conversely, if you tend to have higher blood glucose levels, you might want to inject into your abdomen, which will absorb it more quickly.

Needles/sharps disposal

If you use needles and syringes, you should participate in a local or national sharps disposal program. Needles and lancets should not be tossed away in the trash like the rest of your garbage because

Other Insulin Tips

- Don't ever use insulin that is or has been frozen. Throw it out.
- Sometimes insulin leaks out a little after being injected. If this happens to you, count to five before withdrawing the needle.
- If you have a tendency to bruise, make sure that you are not injecting too fast, that your insulin is at room temperature, that you have a short needle, and that you are rotating injection sites.
- Wash your hands before injecting! Alcohol is generally not needed to wipe the skin unless it is dirty or covered with lotion.
- Always carry a back-up bottle of insulin so you never get caught short.
- Insert the needle straight in at a 90° angle.
- If you are mixing insulin in one syringe (but never glargine or detemir), start with the clear one and go to cloudy. If you miscalculate, throw it away and start over.
- Where there is air in the syringe, there is no insulin. A little air won't hurt you, but it does mean you are not getting the full dose of insulin. If you see an air bubble, either tap it out or, if you are dealing with one type of insulin, push it rapidly back into the vial and the bubble should go away.
- Adjust insulin doses under the guidance of your health care provider.

Glucagon: Overdraft Protection against Severe Lows

An injectable form of glucagon is your first aid kit in the event of severe hypoglycemia, when you cannot administer your own 15 grams of carbohydrate. Glucagon is a hormone naturally produced by the alpha-cells in the pancreas. When glucose is low, glucagon is released and tells the liver to release glucose.

If you are on insulin and have ever had a blood glucose level less than 45 mg/dl, you should have a glucagon injection kit and show your family or friends how to use it. When glucagon is injected, it quickly raises blood glucose levels to bring you out of unconsciousness. It's common to feel nauseated or vomit immediately after awakening from a glucagon injection. Because the raise in glucose caused by glucagon is short lived, you must immediately ingest some form of carbohydrate, such as glucose gel or juice.

they might poke someone who handles the trash. If you're lucky, your community may have a sharps container pick-up service or drop-off center. Call your waste management company to find out what options are near you. There are also some national mail-back services that are either independent (check your local pharmacy) or associated with a syringe and needle manufacturer, such as BD (www.bd.com/sharps).

PERSONAL GOAL

This week (date _____), I decided I can (*check one*):

☐ Start a new vial of insulin if I suddenly see an increase in my blood glucose levels.

☐ Do not take rapid- or short-acting insulin until I am ready to eat.

☐ Roll my NPH (cloudy) insulin vial or pen prior to using it.

☐ Take my glargine or detemir about the same time every day.

☐ On my calendar, mark the expiration dates for insulin vials or pens after I open them.

☐ Keep unopened insulin vials in the refrigerator and opened ones at room temperature.

☐ Check the expiration date on my insulin.

☐ Call my local waste management company to find out about local needle disposal regulations.

☐ Other: _____.

🙂 **I'm insulin resistant. I'm resistant to taking insulin.**

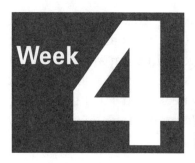

Week 4

Pause for Podiatry

The first step toward foot health is a visit with a foot care specialist (a podiatrist). A podiatrist will check the sensitivity of your feet with a monofilament (a harmless piece of plastic) and a tuning fork. You may also have a Doppler test (a painless in-office ultrasound) screening for peripheral arterial disease (PAD) and X-rays to check for bone problems. Your podiatrist can trim your nails to prevent them from becoming ingrown, thin down thick nails, and provide custom footwear (orthotics) designed to reduce pressure and foot pain.

Do I need to see the podiatrist if I'm not having problems?

Yes, but it doesn't have to be a podiatrist, just someone who specializes in foot care. Diabetes puts you at a risk for foot problems. When blood glucose levels are high for months on end, the nerves going to your feet can lose their ability to detect pain, heat, cold, and pressure. If you can't feel in your feet and get a cut, blister, or callus, you may not know it. If you have circulation problems, healing becomes difficult, and if your blood glucose level is elevated, bacteria will thrive. Even a small break in the skin can turn into a terrible infection under these circumstances. The key to good health is to be hypervigilant in regard to your foot care, to quickly detect foot problems, and to see a podiatrist.

Do Any of These Apply to You?

If any of the following do, then you should make an appointment with a podiatrist as soon as possible.

- Do you have an open wound? (Get to the doctor today. It can save a limb.)

- Do you have a corn, blister, or callus?
- Are there any red spots on your foot?
- Do your feet have a strong odor?
- Are your feet cold most of the time?
- Are you able to cut your own toenails?
- Are your toenails thick, jagged, or ingrown?
- Is the skin between your toes cracked?
- Do you have deep cracks in the skin of your feet?
- Do you have numbness, tingling, or pain?
- Do your feet kill you at the end of the day or keep you up at night?
- Is one of your feet hot and the other not?

PERSONAL GOAL

This week (date _____), I decided I can (*check one*):

☐ Make an appointment with a foot care specialist (call immediately if I have open wounds, hot spots, redness, or swelling in my feet or fever or chills).

☐ Check the American Podiatric Medical Association's website for podiatrists in or near your area at www.apma.org and call my insurance company about coverage for a podiatrist.

☐ Get a peripheral arterial disease (PAD) screening test if I'm over 50 or have leg pain or cramping.

☐ Give away a least one pair of uncomfortable shoes in my closet and one worn-out pair of socks from my drawer.

☐ Quit smoking to reduce my risk for foot problems.

☐ Get a mirror to check the bottom of my feet and apply lotion to my heels every day.

☐ Go to a specialist for treatment on an ingrown toenail.

☐ Other: _____.

My little toe has a corn, and my big one has a cauliflower.

Work Yourself Sick

 Do you have a lot of job-related stress? If you do, you need to learn how to manage it. People with high levels of work-related stress have 50% more health care expenses, according to a National Institute of Occupational Safety and Health report. Your ability to handle work stress can affect your diabetes management.

Stress on the job comes from ourselves (our personalities and work habits) and the work environment (support from peers and management, job expectations, work hours, and physical demands). We work hard, work for longer hours, and have crazy commutes. One study found that people who had shorter commutes and lower salaries were happier and less stressed than those with longer commutes and higher salaries. The time not spent on commuting allowed time for extra sleep, relaxation, and connecting with friends.

Techniques to De-stress Your Work Life

- **Turn gripes into gratitude**. Complaining is commonplace, so turn it around and look for the positives. Replace "I had the worse day ever" with "The best thing that happened to me today was . . ." Look for things that bring you joy.
- **Beat the clock**. Running late to work can stress out anyone. Turn that situation around by leaving early for work, so you'll have time to leisurely commute. Look around as you go to work; you'll see things you never saw for years.
- **Organize, don't agonize**. Tackle that tough assignment first and you won't spend days obsessing over deadlines. Budget time for projects like you would your money for household bills. Get a spending plan—for your work time. Prioritize and evaluate your goals every day.
- **Manage your technology time**. Do checking e-mail and answering the phone get you off track? Set up a general schedule to check e-mails at the start of your day, midway through, and an hour before leaving. Manage your phone time by screening calls. Return calls before lunch or close to quitting time to keep conversations short.

- **One pile at a time**. Multitasking can be great, but it's a problem if you never get anything done and that stresses you out. Make an effort to take a deep breath and tackle projects one at a time, if you can.
- **Take a break**. Get away from the work. Go get a glass of water or a cup of tea. Find a few minutes to close your eyes and visualize your favorite getaway. Find a friend and drag him or her to a coffee break. Get outside and take a short walk.
- **Stash healthy snacks.** People who are stressed out tend to eat to cope with that stress. People who experience job-related stress are 73% more likely to become obese. Instead, stock up on healthy desk snacks, so your blood glucose stays level.
- **Find the funny.** Surround yourself with people who are willing to laugh. Share humorous anecdotes. Be playful. Be goofy. Surround yourself with something that'll make you smile during the workday.
- **Be gentle and kind to yourself.** Cut yourself some slack. Learn as you go. Don't add to your work burden by giving yourself grief. Learn to take responsibility for those issues that are under your control; for those that you can't control, it's not really worth the stress.
- **Beware of burnout.** If you dread going to work, feel like you are just going through the motions, or are checking out mentally, try to take a day off from work. Your mental health will thank you.

PERSONAL GOAL

This week (date _____), I decided I can (*check one*):

☐ Put in that long overdue request for a vacation.
☐ Identify three good things that happened every day this week.
☐ See a therapist.
☐ Take a daily break.
☐ Block off time to finish that one project that's been nagging me.
☐ Buy an assortment of tasty healthy snacks.
☐ Find someone to laugh with every day.
☐ Other: _____.

 Hmm. When was the last time I took a sick day?

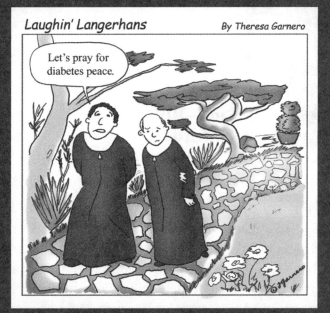

Month 6

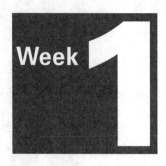

Week 1

Salt and Safety

History of salt

Salt is ancient. It's a common mineral collected from dried-out lakes (rock salt) or extracted from seawater (sea salt). As early as 4,000 years ago, people knew that salt helped preserve food, making it an extremely valuable commodity. Salt used to be in short supply and expensive because of the work needed to process and transport it. Salt has caused wars, invasions, and mass movements in the human population. The power of salt lingers in our language, too. The Latin word for "salt" is *sal*. Roman soldiers were believed to have been paid with salt, which was called a *salarium* in Latin. We call this a "salary." Fast forward to your table.

Halt the salt.

Before you reach for the saltshaker or a packaged food that has enough sodium to rid your neighborhood of snails, think over some of these facts:

- Most people in the U.S. take in twice as much sodium as is recommended, between 4,000 to 5,000 mg/day instead of the recommended maximum of 2,300 mg/day.
- One teaspoon of salt has 2,300 mg of sodium.
- Some people are more sensitive to sodium than others: people with hypertension, African Americans, and middle aged and older adults.
- Over 75% of dietary sodium comes from processed or packaged foods.
- Decreasing sodium intake can decrease blood pressure.

- More than two out of every three people with diabetes also have high blood pressure.
- Increasing the amount of potassium in your diet can reduce the effects of sodium on blood pressure.

How to Shove that Salt Away

- Use fresh produce or frozen and canned items without added salt.
- Eat fresh fish, poultry, and lean meats instead of canned or smoked meats or cold cuts.
- Retire your saltshaker.
- Buy products that are salt free, sodium free, or low in sodium.
- Check food labels and choose brands that are lower in sodium.
- Read over-the-counter medication labels (some, like antacids and stool softeners, contain a lot of sodium).
- Go for cooked dry beans instead of canned beans.
- Rinse canned foods (vegetables, beans, and tuna) to remove some of the salt.
- Pick unsalted nuts and seeds over the salted varieties.
- Consider using a salt substitute, but check with your doctor first.
- Eat at least 4,700 mg of potassium a day (fruits and veggies are full of potassium).

Season with spices instead.

Discover the incredible flavors that spices have to offer. You may find that salt was a boring waste of time once you set foot into the rich world of herbs. Try some of these sumptuous alternatives and bring the exotic flavors of the world into your diet.

For meat, poultry, and tofu: allspice, basil, caraway seeds, cilantro, chives, curry powder, dill, dry mustard, garlic, ginger, lemon or lime juice, nutmeg, onion, paprika, turmeric, parsley, sage, rosemary, thyme

For fish: basil, curry powder, dill, garlic, lemon or lime juice, dry mustard, nutmeg, paprika, parsley, rosemary, sage, turmeric

For vegetables: cider vinegar, dill, garlic, dry mustard, dried oregano, lemon thyme, dried basil, onion, paprika, pimiento, rosemary, Italian seasoning, cilantro, sage

For salads: basil, caraway seeds, chives, cider/red wine or other flavored vinegar, cilantro, dried oregano, Italian seasoning, lemon or lime juice, onion, paprika, parsley, pimiento

For soups: basil, caraway seeds, chives, cilantro, curry powder, dried oregano, Italian seasoning, onion, paprika, parsley, cilantro

For fruit: allspice, almond extract, cinnamon, ginger, nutmeg, peppermint extract

For sauces: basil, chives, dill, dry mustard, paprika, parsley, rosemary, cilantro, turmeric

---

PERSONAL GOAL

This week (date ____), I decided I can (*check one*):

☐ Taste my food before adding salt.
☐ Try a sodium-free dried spice during a meal rather than salt.
☐ Add up how much sodium I eat in a day.
☐ Choose low-sodium foods that contain no more than 140 mg of sodium per serving.
☐ Throw a retirement party for the saltshaker.
☐ Ask my pharmacist about the sodium content of my prescription and over-the counter medications (and for low-sodium alternatives). I won't stop my medication without my health care provider's advice.
☐ Other: _____.

Gone are the days of innocence... and salt.

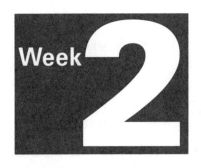

Week 2

The "Work" in Workout

What's the best exercise?

The best exercise is the one that you're most likely to do and enjoy on a regular basis. When choosing an exercise, think about your goals (weight loss, good health, participate in a team sport, or training for a competition), your interests, and your schedule. If you love skiing but live in the desert, then you're not going to be doing it consistently, even if you love it. The ideal exercise program will include cardiorespiratory endurance, muscular strength, muscular endurance, and flexibility. Let's review:

Cardiorespiratory endurance. This is your body's ability to deliver oxygen and nutrients during periods of nonstop, aerobic (oxygen-requiring) exercise, preferably for at least 20 minutes or longer, done at least three times a week. Examples include brisk walking, jumping rope, cycling, rowing, swimming, cross-country skiing, figure skating, rollerblading, and jogging.

Muscular strength. This is your muscles' ability to exert force for a brief amount of time. The prime example is weight lifting.

Muscular endurance. This is your muscles' ability to sustain repeated contractions, preferably done at least three times a week. Some examples include weight training for all the muscle groups, calisthenics, push-ups, and sit-ups.

Flexibility. This is your muscles' and joints' ability to move through a full range of motion. For example, sitting and reaching toward your toes measures the flexibility of your lower back and hamstrings (the back part of your upper legs).

How hard should I exercise?

You should work hard enough to get your body above its resting level. Follow a regular workout schedule at least three times a week to see effects. Avoid consecutive days of hard exercise or a string of consecutive days or weeks with no exercise at all. If you fall off the exercise wagon, every day is a new opportunity to start again.

Follow your heart...rate. Your heart will tell you if the workout is intense enough to get you positive effects. Exercise that doesn't push your heart rate up to 70% of its maximum and keep it there for 20 minutes will not contribute significantly to your fitness level. If your goal is to lose weight, you'll need to keep your target heart rate between 60 and 70% at least five days a week. Target heart rates differ, so consult with your health care provider before beginning an exercise program.

You can find your target heart rate by looking at the following chart:

Age	Target Heart Rate Zone
20 years	100–150 beats per minute
25 years	98–146 beats per minute
30 years	95–142 beats per minute
35 years	93–138 beats per minute
40 years	90–135 beats per minute
45 years	88–131 beats per minute
50 years	85–127 beats per minute
55 years	83–123 beats per minute
60 years	80–120 beats per minute
65 years	78–116 beats per minute
70 years	75–113 beats per minute

How do I check my pulse?

Use the index and middle fingers of your dominant hand (your right hand if you're right-handed) to feel the area inside your wrist on your non-dominant hand below the base of your thumb (your left hand, if you're right-handed). Count your heart beats for 10 seconds and multiply that by 6 to get the beats per minute. The next time you see your pharmacist or health care provider, have them teach you how to check your pulse. If you're feeling particularly modern, you can also buy a heart rate monitor (such as a Polar heart rate monitor, www.polarusa.com, or one from Omron, www.omronhealthcare.com)

PERSONAL GOAL

This week (date _____), I decided I can (*check one*):

- ☐ Push myself to exercise harder. No one else can do it for me.
- ☐ Put together a hot playlist or mixtape for my cardio workouts.
- ☐ Slow down if I cannot carry on a conversation while exercising.
- ☐ Calculate my target heart rate.
- ☐ Ask my health care provider to show me how to take my pulse.
- ☐ Stop exercising if I have chest pain, severe shortness of breath, or leg pain and call my health care provider immediately.
- ☐ Inject insulin into an area that I won't use for exercise (e.g., if going running, don't inject into legs).
- ☐ Increase the intensity, frequency, and duration of my exercise activities.
- ☐ Other: _____.

Scooping ice cream is an effective muscular strengthening technique.

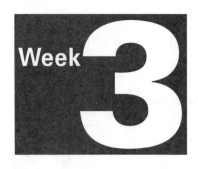

Week 3

Finding Insulin Harmony

This week will focus on insulin delivery and strategies used to fine tune insulin dosage. This overview is not intended to replace the individualized care you need to receive from your health care provider. But you can use this information as a starting point to discuss options with whoever prescribed your insulin.

Delivery options

We have come a long way from glass syringes with hand-sharpened needles and injections of thick, brown solutions made from ground-up cow pancreases that required injecting well over twenty times the amount of insulin than is used today. Technology now offers people with diabetes many insulin-delivery systems.

Syringe and vial. This was the first insulin-delivery system available and is the most common way to take insulin. It is usually the most economical, too. You manually draw up the insulin and inject it yourself.

Insulin pens. This is a popular, easy-to-use option with self-contained insulin in the shape of a small pen. Insulin pens offer a convenient way to carry and discretely use insulin in public. Be sure to "prime" the pen (also known as an "air shot") by discarding two units into the trash (or according to the manufacturer's guidelines). This makes sure you will get the full dose by eliminating any spaces of air in the system. Also, after the needle is inserted, push down *firmly* on the plunger for three to five seconds to be certain you get the full amount. Some systems display large, easy-to-read dosages; others include a clicking sound to indicate the number of units dialed up, which makes them suitable for people with vision problems. *Warning to left-handed* *people:* be careful to read the units correctly. You could accidentally take nine units instead of six units with some systems because the numbers will be reversed when using your left hand.

Insulin pumps. Pumps continuously deliver insulin through a device about the size of a pager and a tiny, plastic tube inserted under the skin. It has revolutionized the way in which diabetes is managed. The benefits include fewer injections (because you only change the plastic tube, or catheter tubing, every two to three days) and improved freedom from rigid schedules. The disadvantages are the initial intensive training required to properly use the device and the necessity to check glucose levels 6–10 times a day.

Needle-free injectors. This is perhaps the least known method of insulin delivery. The device looks similar to an insulin pen, only wider, and instead of a needle, it uses a high-pressure mechanism that delivers a fine spray of insulin through the skin. Insurance coverage for these handy, but expensive, devices varies.

Inhalable insulin. This was the latest insulin breakthrough, allowing patients to breathe in short-acting insulin through a tube-like dispenser. It was released in 2006 but withdrawn from the market in late 2007 because not many people were using it. Other plans have been in the pipeline, so inhalable insulin may still be available in the future, but not right now.

What is the best syringe?

The answer to this question is different for every individual, but three components to making your decision are syringe size, needle width, and needle length.

Size. Syringes come in three basic sizes: 1 cc (holds up to 100 units), 1/2 cc (holds up to 50 units), and 3/10 cc (holds up to 30 units). Make sure your syringe can hold slightly more than the amount of insulin you are taking; this makes it easy to see how much insulin you are getting. Most syringes have one-unit measurements. A few brands offer half-unit or two-unit measurements.

Length. You'll also need a needle length that's suitable to your body type. Needles are available in short—five-sixteenths of an inch

(8 mm)—and standard—half-inch (12.7 mm)—lengths. If your weight is ideal, use the short needle. If you have extra padding, a standard-sized needle is probably more appropriate.

Width. Manufacturers offer several gauges (needle width or thickness) to provide a more comfortable injection. You can find needle gauges of 28, 29, 30, and 31 (the higher the gauge number, the thinner the needle thickness).

Can I reuse my insulin syringes?

Can you or should you? It's generally best to never reuse a syringe. The needles are so fine that, on a microscopic level, the needle tip bends with reuse and causes tissue damage and pain. The other risk is that you can contaminate your insulin bottle by not using a sterile needle (do *not* attempt to clean *any* needle or lancet with an alcohol wipe, as this will only introduce bacteria and might remove the protective coating intended to reduce pain). It is especially dangerous to reuse a needle if you use two types of insulin because that will contaminate your insulin bottles. And never reuse an insulin pen needle because the device may not function properly and you might dose incorrectly.

PERSONAL GOAL

This week (date _____), I decided I can (*check one*):

☐ Have my health care provider double check my insulin-delivery technique.

☐ Check with my pharmacist or certified diabetes educator about the best syringe for me.

☐ Ask to see an insulin pen.

☐ Other: _____.

**No inhalable insulin?
But I want my insulin bong!**

Higher Ground

 People frequently underestimate the power that spirituality can bring to their health and wellness, regardless of the form in which that spirituality presents itself. Some examples include faith-based practices (going to church or temple, praying, watching your favorite minister on TV, reading scripture, etc.), meditating, being one with nature, journaling, or volunteering. Some religious affiliations offer group diabetes education and support.

Stepping outside of oneself offers positive benefits for diabetes self-management because it can reduce stress levels. We often get caught up in the grind of daily life. Take the time to step away and do something good for your soul.

Have you tried walking a labyrinth? They are usually set up outdoors and have paths that twist and turn to the center and then head back out toward the exit. Walking a labyrinth offers you a way to quiet your mind and awaken your inner wisdom. Many churches, schoolyards, and community centers have them. You can even make your own (see www.labyrinthproject.com).

Other helpful ideas are listed here. Choose at least three that resonate with you that will be your focus for the week.

PERSONAL GOAL

This week (date _____), I decided I can (*check one*):

☐ Develop my own healing rituals.
☐ Find delight in paradox.
☐ Ask people about themselves.
☐ Lighten up on those closest to me.
☐ Spend some quiet time out in the fresh air.
☐ Other: _____.

 I'm not lost, just walking a mental labyrinth.

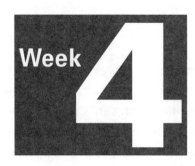

Week 4

Achoo! The Flu and You

What's the fuss over the flu?

When the flu enters the picture and you have diabetes, your chances of getting seriously ill are much greater than those of the general population. If you get the flu, you can face complications, potential hospitalization, and, much worse, death. An ounce of prevention can save your life. Getting the flu shot and frequently washing your hands during flu season are the best ways to reduce your chances of catching the flu.

When should I get vaccinated?

As long as your health care professional has cleared you for a flu shot, you should probably get it during the fall. If you miss that window, find out if it's okay to get one later because the flu season can last into spring. Encourage family members to get vaccinated, too.

Where can I get a vaccination?

You can get one from your health care provider and sometimes at local health fairs.

Helpful Prevention Reminders

- Avoid exposure to the flu by staying away from people who are ill.
- Wash your hands regularly, even obsessively.
- Build your resistance and ability to fend off illness by eating healthfully, staying fit, and getting plenty of rest.
- Stay home if you are sick.
- Make sure that your health care professionals are also washing their hands. If you didn't see them wash their hands, ask if they did.
- Cover your mouth and nose when sneezing or coughing.

PERSONAL GOAL

This week (date _____), I decided I can (*check one*):

☐ Stay away from people who are sick.
☐ Wash my hands frequently.
☐ Get the flu vaccination if it's fall or mark my calendar to remind myself to have one.
☐ Encourage my family members to get the flu vaccination and, if they do get sick, encourage them to take flu medications within two days of becoming ill.
☐ Clean my work area (phone and keyboard) with antiseptic wipes.
☐ If I get the flu, stay hydrated, check my blood glucose every couple of hours, and call my health care provider.
☐ Avoid smoking or being exposed to secondhand smoke to increase my resistance to illness.
☐ Get at least seven hours of sleep for five nights.
☐ Other: _____.

I got the flu the same time my parakeet got the avian flu.

What a Pain

 When is the last time you had pain? Are you in pain right now? If you haven't witnessed it firsthand, pain— whether short or long term—can raise blood glucose levels. The body responds to the stresses of pain by releasing epinephrine, the fight-or-flight hormone that ultimately raises blood glucose levels. Epinephrine has this effect because deep down in your instincts, it thinks you'll need that extra fuel to fight a tiger or run away from danger. With pain, this response is lessened but still in effect.

Pain interferes with everyday life. Chronic pain affects a person's ability to perform diabetes self-care behaviors, especially when it comes to healthy eating, being active, and taking medications. When pain continues over time, a person may avoid activities out of fear of increased pain and become less active, limit social encounters, and withdraw from other life activities. Pain is also often associated with depression.

How is pain diagnosed?

Pain is subjective, so no two people have the same description of their pain. It doesn't show up on an MRI or a blood test. People can look fine and be in pain, that's why a pain-rating scale is commonly used to determine severity of pain. The scale is from 0 to 10, with 0 being "no pain" and 10 being "the worst pain ever." This helps keep you and your health care provider on the same page when discussing pain. If you say "my pain is a 7 out of 10," you will get your message across more clearly than by saying "my pain is tolerable."

Breaking away from pain

As pain persists, people can develop negative thoughts about themselves (e.g., "I'm worthless because I can't support my family") and negative beliefs about their pain experience (e.g., "Nothing will help this get better"). These feelings, coupled with decreased enjoyment in life, can lead to distress and depression. Ending this association of pain and depression may require the use of medication (painkillers) and cognitive behavioral therapy (a method of dealing with the negative thoughts typically related to pain; you'd need to meet with a medical social worker for this therapy).

PERSONAL GOAL

This week (date _____), I decided I can (*check one*):

☐ Initiate a conversation about any pain I am experiencing.

☐ Report pain to my health care provider using the 0 to 10 scale, with 0 being "no pain" and 10 being "the worst pain ever."

☐ See a medical social worker who can help me learn to use cognitive behavior therapy.

☐ Note pain levels in my blood glucose logbook to identify trends.

☐ Take my painkiller medication before my pain is severe.

☐ Write down any negative thoughts I have about pain.

☐ Come up with a positive mantra and start using it daily to cope with frequent pain (my pain is less today, look at what I can do, I am at peace, etc.).

☐ Ask about seeing a pain specialist.

☐ Other: _____.

Diabetes is a pain in the pancreas.

MONTH 6: REVIEW

Today's date: _____

You started this journey of diabetes self-discovery about six months ago. What have you learned?

Look back over the first six months and review all of the goals you made for yourself. While you review, keep the following questions in mind:

What worked? _____

_____

What didn't? _____

_____

What would you do differently? _____

_____

Go back and identify at least five new goals (from day 1 through month 6) that you would like to try:

1. _____

2. _____

3. _____

4. _____

5. _____

Update the status of each of your self-care areas.

Before meal blood-glucose level averages_____ mg/dl
Two-hour after-meal blood glucose level averages
_____ mg/dl
(Before meal target is 70–130 mg/dl; 2 hours after meals is less than 180 mg/dl.)

Last A1C test result? _____ %
(Target: less than 7%)

Last blood pressure reading _____ mmHg
(Target: less than 130/80 mmHg)

When was the last time you talked with your health care provider about your blood pressure? _____

What was your highest blood glucose level?_____mg/dl
The lowest? _____mg/dl Why? _____

How confident do you feel about meal planning and carbohydrate counting for managing your diabetes? Circle one:
    very confident   somewhat confident   not confident
If you do not feel you have a solid grasp on what to eat, please see a registered dietitian and certified diabetes educator to get the answers.

Over the past several months, how many days a week on average did you exercise?
☐ 5+ days/week
☐ 3–4 days/week
☐ 1–2 days a week
☐ None
☐ I am unable to exercise

Do you feel better equipped to deal with the reality of your diabetes diagnosis? Why or why not? _____

Did you take your medication on time?

Circle one: Nearly always   Sometimes   Almost never

Have you identified humorous situations in everyday moments? Do these help to lighten the burden of diabetes self-care? _____

_____

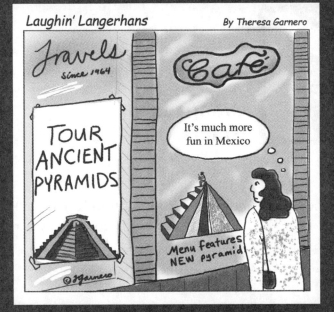

Month 7

Week 1

Orange Is for Grains

The U.S. Department of Agriculture's new MyPyramid provides a customized approach to healthy eating and exercise based on one's age, sex, and activity. The former pyramid had a "one size fits all" approach, had vague descriptions about serving sizes, and nothing about exercise.

The new pyramid shows food groups as a series of colors. The bands of colors are in different widths to represent how much of a particular food someone should eat in a day. The colors are orange for grains, green for vegetables, red for fruit, yellow for fats and oils, blue for dairy, and purple for meats and beans. Over the course of the next several months, we will review each section.

Let's talk about grains.

A grain is the small, dry, one-seeded fruit of a cereal grass in which the fruit and the seed walls are united. Foods made from wheat, rice, oats, barley, and cornmeal, including bread, cereals, pasta, oatmeal, cereals, tortillas, and grits, are examples of grain products.

- **Whole grains** contain the entire grain kernel (the bran, germ, and endosperm) and include whole-wheat flour, whole-wheat bread or crackers, cracked wheat (bulgur), oatmeal, brown rice, wild rice, whole cornmeal, whole rye, buckwheat, popcorn, and whole-wheat pasta. At least half of your grains should be whole grains.
- **Refined grains** have been processed to remove the bran and germ. Unfortunately, this process also removes a lot of the parts of the grain that are good for you, including the bran, iron, and many B vitamins. Refined grains have a finer tex-

ture and shelf life and include white flour, white bread, white rice, most pastas, muffins, couscous, flour and corn tortillas, noodles, grits, and pretzels.

How much grain should I eat in a day?

Have at least 6 ounces of grain every day and at least half of those (3 ounces) should come from whole grains (1-ounce examples: 1/2 cup of cooked pasta, rice, or cereal; about 1 cup of breakfast cereal; or 1 slice of bread). Grains contain carbohydrate, so you should watch your serving sizes.

PERSONAL GOAL

This week (date _____), I decided I can (*check one*):

☐ Choose foods that have one of the following whole-grain ingredients listed first on the ingredient list: whole grain, whole wheat, whole oats, whole rye, wild rice, brown rice, graham flour, oatmeal, whole-grain corn, or bulgur.
☐ Replace refined grains with whole grains.
☐ Try brown or wild rice in place of white rice.
☐ Bake some stuffed peppers with a brown rice and mushroom stuffing.
☐ Add barley to soup or stews.
☐ Cook up brown or wild rice ahead of time to have it available as a quick side dish.
☐ Try a whole-grain snack chip.
☐ Have popcorn for a snack without the salt and butter.
☐ Other: _____.

 The same year the new food pyramid was released, the grain industry moved to Orange County.

Celebrations

Parties can pose a challenge for people with diabetes. Birthdays, anniversaries, holidays, and other celebrations present a minefield of situations that people with diabetes will have to navigate. With just a little planning, you can prevent turning a joyous occasion into a health care calamity.

Discuss your individual approaches to holidays and celebrations with your diabetes health care team (especially when it comes to alcohol; remember, practice moderation and take it with food). Keep your blood glucose monitor handy and check it periodically at any event, as that's the only way to know if you are safe or headed for trouble.

Birthdays

If cake is important, please have *some*. You can exercise earlier in the day or after the dessert, adjust the carbs for your meal, or prepare extra diabetes medication, if needed. Birthdays are special events, so you shouldn't be punished or deprive yourself just because you have diabetes. You can also try an activity that doesn't involve food (such as shopping, going to the movies or the theater, playing games, making out).

Holidays

- **New Year's Eve (December 31).** You may need less basal evening insulin should you have champagne on December 31. This can help prevent starting the New Year with hypoglycemia. Carry emergency glucose tablets and a protein bar. You might try a small snack before arriving at a party so you can avoid all-night grazing.
- **Eid al-Adha (the Muslim festival of sacrifice, about 70 days after Ramadan).** Eid al-Adha commemorates Ibrahim's willingness to sacrifice his son for Allah. It concludes with millions of Muslims taking the pilgrimage to Mecca, Saudi Arabia. When sharing two-thirds of your meals with the poor, you will need less insulin and medication due to limited food intake. Consider limiting koftas.

- **Chinese New Year (varies, end of January to mid-February).** Traditions require people to practice various customs that promote prosperity (sharing tangerines or oranges to symbolize abundant happiness) and ward off bad spirits (lighting firecrackers and wearing red). This week-long celebration is filled with all kinds of carbs. Be careful when it comes to the togetherness candy tray. Pace yourself and share money-filled red envelopes instead.
- **Easter (varies, late March to late April).** If you're fasting for church service, you may need to reduce or hold off on your morning diabetes medications (check with your health care provider first); pass on the chocolate bunny ears.
- **Ramadan (Islamic month of fasting, dates change, about 13 days earlier each consecutive year).** People with diabetes are not required or advised to fast. If you wish to fast, get an individualized plan together with your care provider to accommodate the pre-dawn to sunset fast to prevent hypoglycemia, hyperglycemia, and dehydration.
- **Thanksgiving (fourth Thursday of November).** Bring a healthy choice to share, have a little of each dish instead of a lot, build exercise into the day, and ask about the best medicine approach to take.
- **Bodhi Day (Buddha's Enlightenment, December 8).** Choose a small portion of rice and milk, count your carbs, and act accordingly. Consider adding a protein. If meditating for hours, you may need less medicine and a way to prevent dehydration.
- **Virgin of Guadalupe feast day (honors the patron saint of Mexico, December 12).** Adjust medicines to handle the several hours of morning fasting followed with high-carb foods (champurrado, tamales, and sweet bread). You may need less evening insulin or to hold off on your morning medications until you have food and additional fast-acting insulin to cover the extra carbs. Bring a sugar source, so you will be prepared if you start to feel dizzy or low.
- **Hanukkah (Jewish Festival of Lights, various dates, normally eight days in December).** Enjoy the stuffed beef brisket or fowl. Try baking potato latkes instead of frying them. Try challah bread made from whole wheat instead of egg-enriched

yeast, and limit the honey-sweetened desserts. Plan for extra walking or extra medications to combat the extra carbs.

- **Christmas (December 25).** Bring a sugar source with you to church services, as lows can occur in the middle of a service. You can also accept all neighborly gifts of baked goods to share with your friends and family. Have a snack if the main feast is delayed. You may need more bolus insulin to account for the big meal. Ask for donations to be made toward diabetes research rather than giving you a gift.
- **Boxing Day/St. Stephen's Day (December 26, in most cases).** Go easy on buffet lines. Fish around for the dime in the plum pudding and limit the cream. All of the other tips about alcohol and exercise apply here, too!
- **Kwanzaa (African-American/Pan-African celebration, December 26 to January 1).** Have the karamu (yams, sesame seeds, collard greens, and hot peppers) early in the evening if you also plan to celebrate New Year's Eve. Factor the candied yams into your bolus insulin dose. Watch your alcohol intake in the passing of a communal unity cup.

PERSONAL GOAL

This week (date _____), I decided I can (*check one*):

- ☐ Check with my health care provider about adjusting my medications for fasting.
- ☐ Carry glucose tablets and a protein bar.
- ☐ Exercise before a feast.
- ☐ Sample a little and skip the second helpings.
- ☐ Go for the one thing I really want at a buffet line.
- ☐ Politely accept baked gifts and pass them on.
- ☐ Periodically check my blood glucose during celebrations.
- ☐ Other: _____.

When can I send my diabetes on an all-expenses-paid vacation?

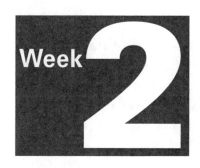

Week 2

Muscle Fitness

Strength training builds muscle mass. Muscles burn more calories than fat, even when you're not exercising. Your muscle fitness helps you maintain or lose weight, manage blood glucose levels, improve balance and posture, and minimize the risk for injury. You can accomplish this through resistance exercises and weight training.

What is resistance training?

Resistance training uses exercises that fatigue the muscles by using your body as a weight (e.g., leg squats and push-ups), by using minimal equipment (e.g., hand weights, jump ropes, elastic bands, balance balls), or by using the machine equipment found in most gyms.

Safety is the first step.

Before you grab those dumbbells, consider the following safety tips:

- Warm up for five minutes by walking on the treadmill, jumping rope, or doing gentle jumping jacks.
- Stretch your muscles when they are warmed up, not cold.
- If you have high blood pressure and are just starting your activity program, only exercise at 50% of your maximum heart rate and gradually build up to 75%.
- Give your muscles one or two days off between strength training exercises (do a different type of activity on alternate days).
- When lifting weights, exhale when lifting or pushing and inhale when lowering or relaxing the muscles.
- Ask your health care provider for an individualized exercise program.

The basics of resistance training

These basics will only skim the surface of resistance training, but should be enough to get you started. Start with an exercise that lets you move in a smooth manner for two sets of ten repetitions with a short rest (about one minute) between sets. Over time, increase the sets to five. When working with weights or exercise equipment that allows you to adjust the tension (such as treadmills, stationary bikes, and stair steppers), begin with the easiest setting or weight. Do the exercise slowly and stay in control of your muscles.

Your mission is to challenge and fatigue your muscles, not pull a muscle or cause a herniated disc. As you get used to resistance training, and with your health care provider's guidance, you can specialize your approach to your personal goals:

- **To increase your muscle strength,** gradually increase the weight and decrease the repetitions (to eight).
- **To increase muscle endurance and toning**, use lighter weights and increase repetitions (up to twenty).

Examples of workout components include the following (get your health care provider's clearance before you dive into any of these):

- Leg squats and side leg raises (two sets of 10 repetitions)
- Wall sit (two sets of 30 seconds)
- Leg lunges with two- to five-pound weights (two sets of 10, each side)
- Bicep curls with no weights or one- to five-pound weights (two sets of 10)
- Torso twists (*gentle* rotations; two sets of 15)
- Leg press at the gym (two sets of 8)
- Bicep curls at the gym (two sets of 8)
- Triceps extensions at the gym (two sets of 8)

PERSONAL GOAL

This week (date _____), I decided I can (*check one*):

☐ Ask my health care provider to review what exercises will work for me.

☐ Give my muscles one or two days off between strength training exercises.

☐ Set the exercise bike on the easiest setting for the next week and increase the resistance for short periods of time.

☐ Challenge my muscles.

☐ Gradually increase weights to build muscle strength.

☐ Do two sets of 10 leg lunges on each leg for the next four days.

☐ Other: _____.

My muscles are giving me a fit.

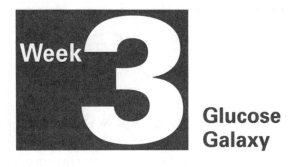

Week 3

Glucose Galaxy

 How high is too high for glucose? There are various degrees of high, but in this section we'll cover two conditions that can arise when blood glucose hits dangerously high levels: hyperglycemic hyperosmolar nonketotic syndrome (HHNS) and diabetic ketoacidosis (DKA).

What is HHNS?

This tongue-twister of a condition (hyperosmolar hyperglycemic nonketotic syndrome) is a serious condition most frequently seen in those who are older and have type 2 diabetes. HHNS is usually brought on by something else, such as an illness or infection.

In HHNS, blood glucose levels rise, and your body tries to get rid of the excess sugar by passing it into your urine. You make lots of urine at first, and you'll be running to the bathroom nonstop. Later, the urine will become dark and trips to the bathroom will be few and far

Warning Signs of HHNS
- Blood glucose level of more than 600 mg/dl
- Dry, parched mouth
- Extreme thirst (although this may gradually disappear)
- Warm, dry skin that does not sweat
- High fever (over 101°F)
- Sleepiness or confusion
- Loss of vision
- Hallucinations
- Weakness on one side of the body
- If you have any of these symptoms, call someone on your health care team immediately.

between. You may also become very thirsty. At this point, your body is nearing dehydration, so you'll need to drink a lot of fluids. If this process continues, severe dehydration will lead to seizures, coma, and eventually death. HHNS may take days or even weeks to develop, so be prepared to identify the warning signs of HHNS.

How do I avoid HHNS? That's easy! The best way to avoid HHNS is to check your blood glucose levels regularly. With regular checking, you should never see your blood glucose go over 600 mg/dl.

What is DKA?

Diabetic ketoacidosis rarely occurs in people with type 2 diabetes... but it can sometimes. This dangerous condition arises when your body begins burning fat for fuel. This process releases a harmful by-product called ketones, which can poison the blood. DKA can result in coma and death, so if you see any of the warning signs, get help immediately.

How do I prevent DKA? DKA usually arises when you're not getting enough insulin, haven't eaten enough food, or whenever you're having a really bad episode of hypoglycemia. By carefully managing your blood glucose levels, you should be able to avoid this critical condition.

Warning Signs of DKA

- Thirst or a very dry mouth
- Frequent urination
- High blood glucose levels
- High levels of ketones in the urine

After the ones above, other symptoms appear

- Constantly feeling tired
- Dry or flushed skin
- Nausea, vomiting, or abdominal pain (Vomiting can be caused by many illnesses, not just ketoacidosis. If vomiting continues for more than 2 hours, contact your health care provider.)
- A hard time breathing (short, deep breaths)
- Fruity odor on breath
- A hard time paying attention or confusion

How do I test for ketones? Ketones can be detected in the blood and through the urine. Testing blood is the more precise method for measuring ketones. Urine testing is less reliable but is easily done by dipping a special testing strip of paper into a cup of urine. For people with type 2 diabetes, ketones are typically not checked because it is not a common issue. Your health care team can recommend whether you need ketone testing as part of your safety net.

PERSONAL GOAL

This week (date _____), I decided I can (*check one*):

☐ Ask my health care provider to go over the signs and symptoms of HHNS and DKA.
☐ Figure out my personal risk for developing any of these conditions.
☐ Get into checking my blood glucose regularly.
☐ Other: _____.

🙂 **Lower your ketone of voice!**

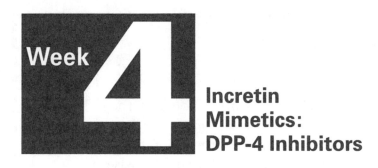

Week 4

Incretin Mimetics: DPP-4 Inhibitors

Who takes this drug?
People with type 2 diabetes are prescribed DPP-4 inhibitors.

What are DPP-4 inhibitors?
Incretin mimetics are a new class of drugs that help the naturally occurring hormones released in the gut to work more efficiently. Dipeptidyl peptidase-4 (DPP-4) inhibitors belong to the class of incretin mimetics and help improve the function of pancreatic beta-cells and control weight. The two primary drugs available in this class are Januvia (sitagliptin) and Galvus (vildagliptin).

How does this drug work?
DPP-4 is an enzyme that affects the levels of the incretin gut hormone called glucagon-like peptide-1 (GLP-1). DPP-4 inhibitors reduce (or inhibit) the amount of DPP-4 produced. By inhibiting DPP-4, GLP-1 levels are allowed to go higher. This is good because increased GLP-1 levels help control blood glucose levels. The higher the blood glucose level, the higher the GLP-1 level should be.

Possible side effects
Upper respiratory tract infections and headaches were rare side effects. More than anything, these drugs may be a pain in your wallet, as they can be quite expensive.

PERSONAL GOAL

This week (date _____), I decided I can (*check one*):

☐ Take my DPP-4 inhibitor within 3 hours of the scheduled dose, if I miss a dose.
☐ Continue to take my medication if my blood glucose is in the target range, unless advised otherwise.
☐ Take my pills as prescribed.
☐ Tell my doctor if I haven't been taking my medication for whatever reason.
☐ Call my doctor to report any sore throat, upper respiratory infection, or severe headache.
☐ Other: _____.

I've got DPP-4 for my GLP-1. Can I buy a vowel?

Eye. Aye, Aye!

Why should I get an eye exam?

Have you had your eyes checked recently? A dilated eye exam is recommended within a few months after being diagnosed with type 2 diabetes and then you should have one annually, regardless of how long you've had diabetes. You may need more frequent exams if you have a condition that requires monitoring.

If you do not have your regular eye check-ups, you are putting yourself at risk of dangerous eye complications and possible blindness. Go see an eye doctor; your eyes will love you for it.

What's the difference between an optometrist and an ophthalmologist?

Both of these specialists can examine your eyes, but only an ophthalmologist can treat retinopathy. Optometrists can check your eyesight and help with minor eye problems, but cannot treat retinopathy. Opticians specialize in eyewear. You may see all three in the course of taking care of your eyes.

My vision isn't great. What's out there to help?

Many resources can assist you if you are living with visual impairment. To begin with, every state has low-vision and blindness agencies that are dedicated to helping you maintain your independence. Specialists can determine the best lighting and magnification products to meet your needs. These include handheld devices, bifocals, large-print reading materials, and computer screen programs that can automatically increase the font size or even describe everything displayed on the screen.

Your diabetes care team can help you get helpful low-vision equipment for diabetes self-management. For example, talking blood glucose meters are available. In addition, manufacturers make syringe magnifiers, needle guides, and vial stabilizers for those who have trouble seeing. Technology can help you learn new ways to stay healthy with diabetes when you have visual impairment.

PERSONAL GOAL

This week (date _____), I decided I can (*check one*):

- [ ] Call and make an appointment for an eye exam.
- [ ] Contact the American Foundation for the Blind at 800-232-5463 for a list of services in my area.
- [ ] Call the National Library Service for the Blind and Physically Handicapped at 888-657-7323 or visit www.loc.gov/nls regarding the postage-free Talking Book Program (has audiobooks and the equipment to play the tapes and texts in Braille).
- [ ] Ask my pharmacist or certified diabetes educator about magnifying devices.
- [ ] Sign up for The Braille Forum, a free monthly publication from the American Council of the Blind (available in most formats) by calling 800-424-8666 or visiting www.acb.org.
- [ ] Other: _____.

I loved my talking meter until it told me to take out the trash.

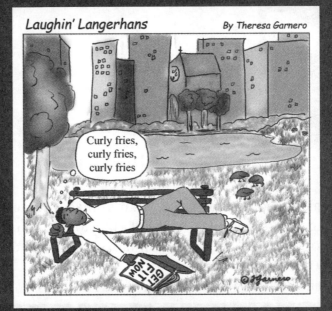

Month 8

Week 1

Green Is for Veggies

This section of the food pyramid makes sense: lots of veggies are green. Do you want a tool to help you manage blood glucose levels and maintain or lose weight? Pile up your plate with nonstarchy veggies!

Here are some of the vegetables and their subcategories.

Dark green	Dry beans and peas (contain carbohydrate)	Orange	Other	Starchy veggies (contain carbohydrate)
Bok choy	Black beans	Acorn squash	Artichokes	Corn
Broccoli	Black-eyed peas	Butternut squash	Asparagus	Green peas
Collard greens	Garbanzo beans	Carrots	Bean sprouts	Green lima beans
Dark green leafy lettuce	Kidney beans	Pumpkin	Beets	Potatoes
Kale	Lentils	Sweet potatoes	Brussels sprouts	
Romaine lettuce	Lima beans		Cabbage	
Spinach	Navy beans		Cauliflower	
Turnip greens	Pinto beans		Celery	
Watercress	Soybeans		Cucumbers	
	Split peas		Eggplant	
	Tofu		Green beans	
	White beans		Green or red bell peppers	
			Iceberg lettuce	
			Mushrooms	
			Okra	
			Onions	
			Parsnips	
			Tomatoes	
			Turnips	
			Wax beans	
			Zucchini	

How many different types of veggies have you consumed this past week? How many of the listed veggies have you not tried? Get creative in finding ways to incorporate more green in your life.

PERSONAL GOAL

This week (date _____), I decided I can (*check one*):

- ☐ Buy in-season vegetables (I'll get the best flavor and they usually cost less).
- ☐ Eat frozen veggies before they get freezer burn.
- ☐ Pay for the convenience of prewashed, precut veggies (cuts down on prep time).
- ☐ Eat a veggie I love.
- ☐ Puree zucchini to add to muffins, French toast, or homemade bread.
- ☐ Make a colorful salad for lunch.
- ☐ Chop up veggie slices and have them ready in the fridge for a healthy snack.
- ☐ Plant a vegetable garden.
- ☐ Other: _____.

 In the Navy...beans.

Incretin Mimetic: Byetta (Exenatide)

Who takes Byetta?
Byetta is prescribed for people with type 2 diabetes.

What is Byetta?
Incretin mimetics are a new class of drugs that help the naturally occurring hormones released in the gut to work more efficiently. Exenatide belongs to this group.

Byetta is the brand name for exenatide and is only administered via injection. Byetta comes in a prefilled pen device and has two available doses: 5 or 10 micrograms (mcg).

How does Byetta work?
Byetta is derived from the saliva of the Gila monster (a slow-moving lizard native to the southwestern U.S.). Don't worry—Byetta is made in laboratories, not taken from lizards, so it's fine for people to use. The lizard's saliva contains a protein called exendin-4, which works like a very important hormone called glucagon-like peptide-1 (GLP-1), but it lasts longer in the body. Both GLP-1 and exendin-4 cause the pancreas to release more insulin in response to meals, which helps control blood glucose levels. Some studies have also shown that Byetta helps some people lose weight or avoid gaining weight. Byetta is known to preserve beta-cell function.

Possible side effects
Nausea is common when the drug is started, but this usually subsides. Hypoglycemia can be a risk if Byetta is used in combination with insulin or pills that cause insulin release (e.g., insulin secretagogues).

Warning
Byetta is not for people with type 1 diabetes. Byetta pens can now be kept at room temperature (but not at more than 77°F) after the first use. Keep unused pens refrigerated at all times (36–46°F). Discard Byetta pens 30 days after first use, even if the pen still has some medication in it. Be sure to rotate injection sites (abdomen, upper arm, and thigh). Do not mix Byetta with insulin.

PERSONAL GOAL

This week (date _____), I decided I can (*check one*):

☐ Inject Byetta anytime within 60 minutes before breakfast and dinner (as prescribed).

☐ Mark on my calendar 28 days after starting a new Byetta pen so I can remember when to start a new one.

☐ Dispose of my used needles according to local laws and regulations.

☐ Report episodes of hypoglycemia or severe nausea to my health care provider.

☐ Other: _____.

 I'm going to get a pet Gila monster, make it mad, and name it Byetta.

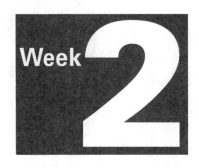

Week 2

Get with the Program: At Home

Have you thought about getting your dose of exercise in the comfort and convenience of your own home? It can be relatively easy to convert a small area in your sweet home into a workout space.

There are benefits to having a home exercise program. It's easier on your wallet, and fewer variables interfere with making it happen (weather, body image concerns, time to commute to the gym, etc.). Household chores are excluded from this segment, unless you spend 30 minutes a day vacuuming until you sweat!

Sounds great, but how do I do it?

Here are two great ways to bring exercise into your own home.

1. Videos. Choose an exercise or activity you enjoy and look for a video to guide you.

- Collage Video is a company that offers every kind of exercise video (VHS or DVD) under the sun, all of which are reviewed by an instructor certified by the American Council on Exercise. Previews and customer reviews of videos are available on their website (www.collagevideo.com).
- Do resistance and low-impact aerobic exercise and stretches with the 45-minute video from Joslin Diabetes Center's Exercise Physiology Department. This cool workout has something for everyone by showing two people, one standing and one sitting down, exercising side-by-side. This great video is called *Keep Moving!...Keep Healthy with Diabetes* and costs around $27.

2. Invest in a home gym. You can get fit if you know the right equipment to buy. Watch out for scams on TV that promise you the world and merely take your hard-earned cash. Do the research to make sure you are getting the right piece of machinery. If you choose this option, be sure to do a lot of research to be sure that you're buying safe, reliable machinery.

PERSONAL GOAL

This week (date _____), I decided I can (*check one*):

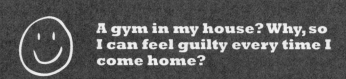

☐ Make a plan to exercise at home.
☐ Lay out my exercise clothes the night before my morning work-out.
☐ Don't buy anything without doing research.
☐ Research a fitness product.
☐ Contact a local gym or exercise equipment store to try out equipment before I buy it.
☐ Find out warranty and return information.
☐ Other: _____.

A gym in my house? Why, so I can feel guilty every time I come home?

The Nerve of Neuropathy

Nerves communicate information about pain, temperature, and touch directly to your brain. If you burn your hand on the stove, your nervous system sends that message at lightning speed to the brain and you pull your hand away without thinking about it. Nerves also help with digestion, bladder function, sexual function, sweating, detection of low glucose levels, and the warning signs of a heart attack.

What is diabetic neuropathy?
Diabetic neuropathy is nerve damage that occurs as a result of uncontrolled blood glucose levels. Neuropathy occurs in nearly half of all people with diabetes and can result in pain or loss of sensation.

How do I know if I really have diabetic neuropathy?
Your health care provider will look at your complete medical picture and may refer you to a neurologist (a doctor who specializes in nerves) for specialized testing. You need a complete physical, blood

What Are the Symptoms of Neuropathy?
- Tingling, burning, or stabbing pains in the feet or hands that is typically worse at night and very sensitive to the touch.
- Very cold or very hot feet or hands.
- Feeling like you are wearing socks or gloves when you aren't.
- Numb or extremely dry feet.
- Weak and unsteady leg muscles.
- Difficulty balancing when walking.
- Frequent indigestion or nausea.
- Vomiting undigested food.
- Feeling bloated or full after very little food.
- Frequent diarrhea or constipation.
- Bladder issues (frequent leakage, infections, urge to go with very little results).
- Sexual problems (trouble getting aroused or reaching orgasm).
- Fast heartbeat while at rest.
- Dizziness when standing.
- No warning signs of low blood glucose.
- Sweating when eating certain foods.

tests, and, depending on your symptoms, X-rays, an ultrasound, and an MRI. The nerve conduction study is the definitive test to prove peripheral neuropathy (in the arms and legs). It is the best test—as long as you come prepared. This is because nerve conduction studies require that small needles be inserted under the skin in numerous places and then a small electrical current is run through your body to test your nerves' reactions. If you're worried about pain, ask your health care provider about taking medication for the pain beforehand.

What are the treatments for diabetic neuropathy?

Preventing the development or progression of diabetic neuropathy through blood glucose control is the first step in treatment. Pain from neuropathy can be debilitating and difficult to manage, so that must also be addressed with a health care provider. Here are some approaches to treatment.

Medication. Many medications help address and minimize the symptoms of neuropathy. Talk with your health care provider about the best one for you because most treatment methods do include a risk of side effects. Options include antidepressants (used in lower doses than those for people with depression), anticonvulsants (reduces the pain of neuropathy), topical creams (sometimes used to treat neuropathy in specific locations), narcotic analgesics (serious painkillers for really bad pain), and anesthetics.

Transcutaneous electrical nerve stimulation (TENS). TENS delivers tiny electrical impulses along specific nerve pathways through small pads placed on your skin. This may help prevent pain signals from reaching the brain. It's safe and virtually painless. Its effectiveness varies based on the type and severity of the neuropathy.

Biofeedback. Biofeedback therapy uses a special machine that teaches you how to control your responses to pain.

Monochromatic infrared therapy (Anodyne therapy). This treatment method uses beams of infrared light to treat neuropathy. The infrared light goes through the skin over the affected area, causes the release of nitric oxide from red blood cells, helps circulation, and improves nerve conduction. Anodyne therapy is covered by many insurance companies, and you can find a physical therapist or physician in your local area who provides this treatment by visiting www.anodynetherapy.com.

PERSONAL GOAL

This week (date _____), I decided I can (*check one*):

☐ Continue checking my blood glucose levels at different times.

☐ Report any symptoms of neuropathy to my health care provider.

☐ Ask my health care provider for help in controlling and managing pain.

☐ Ask my local hospital or medical center about where I can learn about biofeedback techniques.

☐ Ask for a referral to a neurologist.

☐ Other: _____ .

If you have diabetes, sometimes it gets on your nerves.

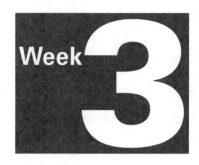

Week 3

Glucose and Blood Pressure Review

 Let's look at the state of your blood glucose and blood pressure levels.

Blood glucose levels

Checking your blood glucose levels has a huge effect on your A1C values, as long as you know what to do with the results.

1. How often do you check?
- ☐ Daily, at varied times (before and two hours after meals)
- ☐ Daily, at one time of the day (e.g., morning only)
- ☐ A few times a week
- ☐ Weekly
- ☐ Rarely
- ☐ My meter isn't working
- ☐ I'm not testing (for whatever reason)
- ☐ Other: _____

2. What is your pre-meal average (more than half of the time)?
- ☐ below 70 mg/dl (see question 3)
- ☐ 71–89 mg/dl
- ☐ 90–130 mg/dl (this is the goal)
- ☐ 131–160 mg/dl
- ☐ 161–190 mg/dl
- ☐ 191–220 mg/dl
- ☐ 221 mg/dl and above

3. How many lows (below 70 mg/dl) have you had this week?
_____.

Call your health care provider if you have more than two readings of less than 70 mg/dl within one week.

4. Most of the time, what is your two-hour after-meal range?
☐ less than 180 mg/dl (this is the goal)
☐ less than 210 mg/dl
☐ less than 240 mg/dl
☐ 241 mg/dl and above

5. If your glucose is not in the target range most of the time or if you are experiencing readings of less than 70 mg/dl more than twice a week, does your health care provider know?
☐ Yes　　☐ No

6. If you have involved your health care provider, has your treatment changed?　☐ Yes　　☐ No

7. If your blood glucose patterns are still outside the target range despite multiple medication adjustments, has your health care provider referred you to a specialist (such as an endocrinologist or a diabetologist)?　☐ Yes　　☐ No

8. What was your last A1C result? _____% (target is less than 7%)　Date taken _____

Blood pressure levels
Time to put the pressure on about bringing your blood pressure down!

1. How often do you check your blood pressure?
☐ Daily, at various times
☐ Daily, in the morning
☐ A few times a week
☐ Rarely
☐ Only at my health care provider's office
☐ I don't have blood pressure monitoring equipment
☐ Other: _____

2. What is your average blood pressure reading?

Systolic (top number)	Diastolic (bottom number)
☐ Less than 130 mmHg (target)	☐ Less than 80 mmHg (target)
☐ 131–140 mmHg	☐ 81–90 mmHg
☐ 141–150 mmHg	☐ 91–100 mmHg
☐ 151–160 mmHg	☐ 101–110 mmHg
☐ 161–170 mmHg	☐ 111–120 mmHg
☐ 171–180 mmHg	☐ 121–130 mmHg
☐ 181 mmHg and above	☐ 131 mmHg and above
☐ Other: _____	☐ Other: _____

3. If you have involved your health care provider, has your blood pressure treatment changed?   ☐ Yes   ☐ No

4. If your blood pressure patterns are still above target despite multiple medication adjustments, has your health care provider referred you to a specialist (such as a cardiologist)?
☐ Yes   ☐ No

PERSONAL GOAL

This week (date _____), I decided I can (*check one*):

☐ Check my blood glucose at times when I normally don't test.

☐ Send my blood glucose data to my health care provider (by fax, e-mail, or phone).

☐ Ask my health care provider for a new treatment plan for problematic blood glucose or blood pressure patterns.

☐ Check my blood pressure at times when I normally don't measure.

☐ Other: _____.

My blood pressure and blood glucose meters chipped in for me to have a massage.

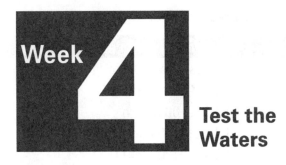

Week 4

Test the Waters

 Test the glucose and jump in—the water's warm! Diabetes does not have to stop you from enjoying activities in or on the water.

Showers, baths, and hot tubs

If you have lost any nerve sensation and cannot feel the difference between hot and cold, test the water temperature on an area that can (like your elbow or wrist). People have burned themselves by getting into a scalding bath or shower (when the water heater thermostat was set at a dangerously high level) because they had lost the ability to feel heat.

Whether you slip into a nice bath or hot tub or want to swim in the pool or with the dolphins, know your blood glucose levels before you start and make sure you have enough fuel to cover your activity. Be prepared and have a stash of supplies to handle lows.

Pools

Check your blood glucose before taking the plunge, swim with others, and have snacks nearby. Follow these precautions and you should be fine.

Oceans, creeks, and rivers

Besides the obvious risks that come with the power of water, beware of potentially harmful concentrations of microorganisms in crowded waters. These parasites and spores are highest when the beaches and rivers are busiest, and they can cause vomiting and diarrhea. If you are not feeling your best, pass on getting into a crowded waterway.

Cruises

Feel like a relaxing vacation cruise? Tell your travel agent you have diabetes when you book your trip. Most cruises offer a wide variety of food choices. Diabetes education cruises will have more sensible cuisine and opportunities to learn ways to manage diabetes (see contact information below).

PERSONAL GOAL

This week (date _____), I decided I can (*check one*):

☐ Check my water heater thermostat and turn it down to a safe level.
☐ Check the water and my blood glucose before I get into a bath or hot tub or go for a swim.
☐ Have juice next to my bath or hot tub in case I feel low.
☐ Book a cruise.
☐ Check out the WAVES (Wellness Adventures: Vacation, Education, Support) Diabetes Program at www.escapesquare.com/waves or call 1-847-917-4277.
☐ Tell a friend about Dialysis at Sea at www.dialysisatsea.com or call 800-544-7604.
☐ Other: _____.

☺ **Surf boards now come in grape glucose tablet flavor, just in case surf's up and my glucose is down.**

Self-Sabotage

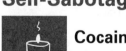

Cocaine/amphetamines

These were popular in the 80s, and they remain deadly in the new millennium. Cocaine and amphetamines can make your blood glucose levels look like a rocket shooting skyward and can be deadly. They put a tremendous amount of stress on your heart and liver. If you do have a habit with these drugs, you need to stop immediately. Find support, beginning with your health care team and support system.

Marijuana

Marijuana use can increase insulin resistance, impair judgment, and give you a case of the munchies, which brings unwanted calories into your diet. Aside from the smoking issue, marijuana use can increase your need for insulin, worsen your blood glucose control due to overeating, and affect your ability to successfully manage blood glucose highs and lows.

Tobacco

Smoking was discussed at length earlier, but it is worth noting again that smoking is dangerous to all people, but doubly dangerous to people with diabetes. If you smoke, get help and support in quitting. If you don't smoke right now, don't start.

PERSONAL GOAL

This week (date _____), I decided I can (*check one*):

☐ Admit I am struggling with a substance abuse
  problem.
☐ Turn down invitations to try a new drug.
☐ Quit smoking (cigarettes, cigars, or joints); quit chewing tobacco.
☐ Drink alcohol with company, and food, only on special occasions.
☐ Say I'm sorry to someone I hurt with my drug-related behavior.
☐ Take a step toward cleaning my body of a toxic addiction.
☐ Check out Alcoholics Anonymous at www.alcoholics-
  anonymous.org or look for a local AA program.
☐ Check out Narcotics Anonymous at www.na.org.
☐ Seek counseling about my prescription drug use.
☐ Other: _____ .

 Do you abuse grapefruit juice?

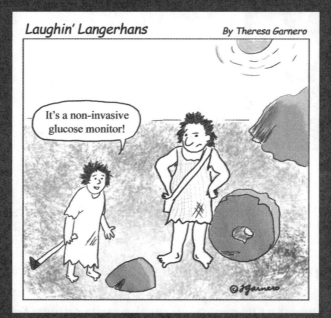

Month **9**

Week 1

Red Is for Fruit

 Mother Nature provides us with this wonderful treat. Fruits are good for you. They're loaded with vitamins and nutrients. You'll do you body and immune system a favor by ignoring the myth that people with diabetes cannot have fruit. It's true! Fruit and diabetes *do* mix, even though they contain carbohydrates—just be sure to count the carb content. Fruits are an essential part of a healthy diet, so make them a part of your lifestyle.

PERSONAL GOAL

This week (date _____), I decided I can (*check one*):

☐ Buy fresh, in-season fruits.
☐ Try something organic or even exotic.
☐ Add chopped-up fruit to my salads.
☐ Keep a bowl of fruit in the kitchen.
☐ Stash a package of dried fruit in my desk.
☐ Barbeque some cubed fruit at a cookout.
☐ Bake an apple or pear for dessert.
☐ Avoid "fruit-flavored" beverages and choose 100% fruit juices.
☐ Other: _____.

 Is the Red Sea one big fruit bowl?

Amylinomimetics:
Symlin (Pramlintide Acetate)

Who takes this drug?
Symlin is prescribed for people with type 1 or type 2 diabetes.

What is Symlin?
The pancreas simultaneously releases the hormones insulin (from the beta-cells) and amylin (from the alpha-cells). Insulin and amylin work together to help control glucose, especially after meals. The synthetic version of amylin is Symlin. Like insulin, Symlin must be injected. *Never mix the two in the same syringe.*

How does Symlin work?
Symlin helps slow digestion, which helps control the rate at which glucose is absorbed into the bloodstream. This in turn reduces appetite and may result in weight loss. It also reduces the glucose released from the liver. Symlin often reduces the amount of insulin that is required by people who inject it. One disadvantage is the increase in number of injections required. The flip side of that, however, is that it can help reduce unpredictable swings in blood glucose levels and improve overall diabetes control.

Possible side effects
Because Symlin lowers blood glucose levels, insulin dosages will need to be reduced or else there is an increased risk of hypoglycemia. Because Symlin slows the rate of digestion, the effectiveness of other medications taken by mouth may be affected.

Warning
Symlin is not recommended for women who are pregnant or breast-feeding.

PERSONAL GOAL

This week (date _____), I decided I can (*check one*):

☐ Ask my health care provider about detailed instructions on how to slowly increase or decrease my Symlin dose.

☐ If I missed my Symlin injection, I won't "make up" the dose. Instead, I'll take my next dose before my next meal.

☐ Skip my Symlin injection if I have hypoglycemia before a meal, if I do not plan to eat, or if I will eat less than 250 calories or less than 30 grams of carbohydrate at a meal.

☐ Skip my Symlin injection if I'm sick and can't eat my usual meal or if I'm going to have surgery or a medical test where I cannot eat beforehand.

☐ Take Symlin and insulin in different devices (insulin syringe or pump) and never mix them.

☐ Inject Symlin in my stomach area (abdomen) or upper leg (thigh), not in my arm.

☐ Take Symlin at room temperature to reduce the possibility of pain or discomfort from the injection.

☐ Store unopened bottles of Symlin in the refrigerator and dispose of any opened vial after 28 days.

☐ Other: _____.

Amy-Lynn...a hormone named after my teenage daughter.

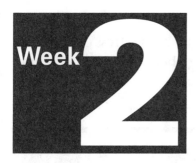

Week 2

Move While You Still Can

The talk of exercise and its benefits can be a downer if you have physical limitations that prevent you from getting regular activity. Whether you have pain, arthritis, weakness from the aftermath of a stroke, or you're unsteady on your feet, chair exercises may be the ticket to increased stamina, muscle strength, and improved blood glucose control.

With a little guidance, you can move your body in a comfortable and effective way to improve flexibility and coordination. You can also do chair exercises while watching TV. Check out the award-winning Armchair Fitness videos that complement each other for a complete fitness program. Ask around for other options in armchair exercises.

PERSONAL GOAL

This week (date _____), I decided I can (*check one*):

- ☐ Visit Armchair Fitness Videos (www.armchairfitness.com).
- ☐ Check out the "Sit and Be Fit" videos from Collage Video by visiting www.collagevideo.com.
- ☐ Ask my health care provider or physical therapist about exercise programs with isometric exercises.
- ☐ Start a short, easy exercise program.
- ☐ Warm up for a few minutes.
- ☐ Do stretching exercises while printing a document, watching TV, or talking on the phone.

- ☐ Sign up for a water exercise program (takes the stress off joints).
- ☐ Note my activity in my logbook to check how it affects my blood glucose.
- ☐ Other: _____.

I've always hated to move, but now I can do it in my chair.

The Skinny on Skin Care

Skin is your personal homeland security system—it protects the body from dangerous environmental elements (bacteria, chemicals, the sun's ultraviolet rays), including heat and cold. It's the largest organ in the body, weighing about 25 pounds, and is one of our most versatile organs.

It functions as a waterproof wrapping for the entire body, regulates body temperature, prevents loss of essential body fluids, and gets rid of toxic substances with sweat. Various skin cells and nerve endings send impulses to the central nervous system and provide the sense of touch. This allows the ability to sense heat, cold, pain, and other sensations. It is also important for general health. If someone is sick, it often shows in the color of his or her skin.

How does diabetes affect my skin?

In the short term, high glucose levels pull water from the skin cells and may cause the skin to be dry or feel itchy or sore. This may lead to cracked skin and worse. A simple scratch or break in the skin can cause an infection. In the long term, high glucose levels can cause the tiny blood vessels near the skin to narrow or even clog, further increasing the risk of infection. Skin problems that are associated with diabetes are numerous and not for the faint of heart. Prevention and early detection of problems is the best treatment.

People with diabetes have higher rates of psoriasis, a condition that affects the skin and joints. Psoriasis causes red, raised areas of dry skin, often seen on the elbows and knees, but can affect any area of skin. Psoriasis can cause arthritis and create an increased risk for heart attacks in people with diabetes. Protect yourself by getting treatment for high blood pressure and high cholesterol and by quitting smoking or reducing your exposure to secondhand smoke.

What can I do to prevent skin problems?

Read through the following list and pick three things to save your skin.

PERSONAL GOAL

This week (date _____), I decided I can (*check one*):

☐ Protect myself from getting minor scratches in my skin (watch out for pets, garden shrubs, long fingernails, splinters) and always wear shoes.
☐ Use mild soap, rinse off thoroughly, and dry myself well (I'll pay attention to places where water likes to hide: under the arms and breasts, the groin area, and between the toes).
☐ Check my skin after each bath or shower to look for any red or sore spots.
☐ Use fragrance-free lotion to keep my skin moist (but not between my toes).
☐ Use a sunscreen daily of at least SPF 15.
☐ Call my skin doctor (dermatologist) for help with any skin issues I'm having.
☐ Wear all-cotton underwear that allows my skin to breathe.
☐ Other: _____.

 With sunscreen, shades, and a helmet, I can finally leave the house.

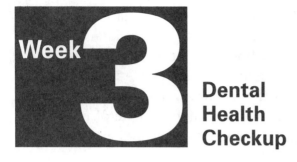

Week **3** Dental Health Checkup

If you've been following along, you'll know that six months have passed and it's time for a dental health checkup.

Answer these questions and then pick a new goal below.

1. How many times did you floss this past week? _____
2. When was the last time you flossed? _____
3. When was the last time you replaced your toothbrush?

   _____

PERSONAL GOAL

This week (date _____), I decided I can (*check one*):

☐ Make an appointment to see my dental hygienist.
☐ Report any tooth or gum problems to my dentist.
☐ Buy products that have the American Dental Association's Seal of Acceptance (meaning the product meets safety and effectiveness standards and that advertising claims are scientifically supported).
☐ Ask my pharmacist if any of my medications could cause dry mouth.
☐ Use lip balm regularly.
☐ Avoid mouthwash with alcohol in it (it may worsen dry mouth).
☐ Rinse my mouth with water immediately after meals.
☐ Ask my dentist about toothpaste specially formulated for dry mouth (e.g., Biotene).
☐ Keep a water bottle handy to moisten my mouth when I need it.
☐ Other: _____.

You've Got Mail...and Strips

Have you thought about getting your diabetes care supplies by mail order? It's a convenient, time-saving option that may also save you money. Many companies offer to bill your insurance, pay for shipping, handle all of the paperwork, ensure your strips/medications don't run out, and provide educational material at no charge. Some are full-service pharmacies that allow you to obtain your medications and products up front without having to pay out of pocket and wait for insurance reimbursement. (If you are ordering insulin by mail, though, be aware of the conditions it may face during shipping—the heat in hot summer months or freezing temperatures in the winter can damage the insulin.) If you're interested, you may want to consider any one of these companies.

PERSONAL GOAL

This week (date _____), I decided I can (*check one*):

☐ Check if my local pharmacy has a mail-order program (and if they will bill my insurance).
☐ Ask my health care provider for a prescription for all diabetes medication and supplies to send to my mail-order company.
☐ See if my health insurance has a mail order provider.
☐ Contact American Diabetic Support Group at 800-830-9211 or visit www.adsgfamily.com.
☐ Contact CCS Medical at 800-726-9811 or visit www.ccsmed.com.
☐ Contact Liberty Medical at 877-542-3610 or visit www.liberty-medical.com.
☐ Contact Medicool, Inc., at 800-433-2469 or visit www.medicool.com.

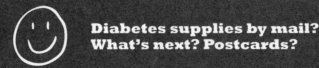

Diabetes supplies by mail?
What's next? Postcards?

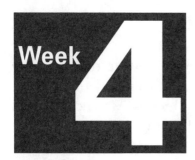

Week 4

Me Time

 When was the last time you did something nice for yourself? Was it this week? This month? Do you do it on a regular basis? We tend to put work, family, and other obligations first, but it shouldn't be that way.

Do you find yourself in a give, give, give mode from dawn until dusk? Try to give yourself just 15 minutes. You're worth it. Ask yourself, "Am I going to let diabetes control me or am I going to make the time to control diabetes?" Check out some ideas on the next page on how to give back to yourself.

PERSONAL GOAL

This week (date _____), I decided I can (*check one*):

☐ Breathe deep and let out a big yawn!

☐ Take a 20-minute nap.

☐ Make an appointment to get a massage for my health, not as a luxury (massage releases neurochemicals that prompt relaxation, which in turn will can lower blood pressure and blood glucose; plus, it feels really good).

☐ Buy a small acupressure roller/foot massaging tool to help me relax and boost my energy.

☐ Listen to my favorite relaxing CD for at least five minutes.

☐ Add a few drops of essential lavender oil to my baths for the calming effects of aromatherapy (try mint, lemon, or pine scents for a refreshing effect).

☐ Schedule time for self-care.

☐ Rent a movie I've been dying to watch, and watch it!

☐ Stand tall.

☐ Other: _____.

☺ **If I can't say nice things to myself, I won't say anything at all!**

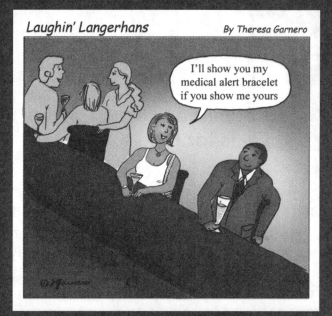

Month **10**

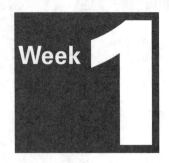

Week 1

Yellow Is for Fat

Don't blink the next time you look at the food pyramid or you'll miss that thin sliver of yellow that represents how much fat and oil we should consume daily—it's the smallest amount of any food group.

Fats were covered closely earlier, but now that it's month 10, it's time to make sure that you're paying attention to the amount of fat in your diet. Choose three of the goals below to further reduce your fat intake. Little steps go a long way in conquering our American obsession with fatty foods.

PERSONAL GOAL

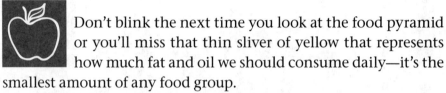

This week (date _____), I decided I can (*check one*):

☐ Trim off any fat from meats.
☐ Avoid fast food for an entire week.
☐ Bake, steam, roast, grill, or broil dishes instead of frying them.
☐ Make an effort to cut down on high-fat foods for the next week or month.
☐ Use lemon or herb seasonings to flavor dishes.
☐ Read food labels for all foods that I buy.
☐ Put away the butter and margarine and find low-fat ways to flavor foods.
☐ Try a vegetarian dish.
☐ Other: _____.

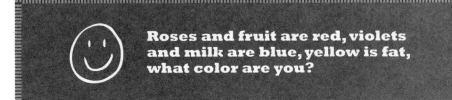

Roses and fruit are red, violets
and milk are blue, yellow is fat,
what color are you?

Eastern Influences:
Meditation, Yoga, and Tai Chi

Meditation

When you meditate, you focus your attention beyond the normal distractions of life. Meditation allows you to relax and improve your quality of life, and it's simple to do! All you need to meditate is to focus on your breathing.

Let's try meditating right now. After you finish reading this paragraph, close your eyes and breathe deeply from your belly. Count four seconds as you slowly inhale and five seconds as you exhale. Focus on your breathing and the present moment. There is no right or wrong way to meditate. All states of consciousness are valuable to your meditation practice whether you focus on breathing, sounds, symbols, colors, or positive thoughts. Allow quiet to enter your mind for just one or two minutes.

Look for everyday opportunities to practice meditation. Try it while walking, standing in line, or while waiting for your computer to boot up. Keep your eyes open and merely focus on your breathing. Or, after a long day, take some time out for an extended period of meditation.

Meditation may not lower your blood glucose like medications, but the peace of mind that it brings to your daily life is priceless.

Yoga

Yoga is the practice of stretching and breathing. Yoga brings the mind and body together through mental, physical, and spiritual aspects of the self. It increases energy, endurance, and flexibility; improves blood pressure, sleep, mood, memory, and balance; and reduces stress. Who wouldn't want all of those benefits?

Before you jump into your favorite yoga pose, take some precautions. Certain postures should be avoided if you have high blood pressure, glaucoma, a herniated disc, or a detached retina. Have a conversation with your health care provider before starting a yoga program.

The best way to learn yoga is to take a basic class or buy a beginner's video. It's generally best to do yoga one or two hours after eating or on an empty stomach (which may put you at risk for hypoglycemia). Be sure to carry your meter and a source of glucose to be safe. Typically, no shoes are allowed in yoga studios, so you'll also need to be extra careful with your feet. Lastly, yoga shouldn't be painful. It's about pushing your muscle resistance without pain or strain. You should stop a pose if you have pain or find yourself holding your breath.

You can then do yoga anytime and anywhere—even at work. Yoga can take just one minute to do and doesn't require a lot of space (yes, 20 minutes is ideal, but don't let that stop you from doing a 60-second exercise here and there). Try any of these:

Chair Pose
From a standing position, inhale and extend straightened arms overhead with palms touching. Bend your knees, lower your buttocks, and angle your torso forward slightly (so it looks like you are about to dive into a pool). Hold the pose for three breaths, exhale, and return to a standing position.

Corpse Pose
This relaxation pose requires that you lie on your back. Relax your physical, mental, and spiritual being by concentrating on your breathing and intentionally relaxing your muscles from head to toe. Rest in this pose for at least 10 minutes.

Easy Pose
A classic meditative pose where you sit with your legs folded, spine straight, and arms relaxed on the knees.

Shoulder Stretches
Raise your hands above your head and inhale. Let your hands gently fold behind your head and exhale. Inhale while you touch the base of your neck with your left hand and you grab your left elbow with your right hand. Stretch the shoulder and exhale. Repeat with right arm.

Squat

Stand with feet apart in a wide stance. Bring your palms together in the middle of your chest. Bend your knees and lower your hips down toward your heels. Press your elbows against the inside of your knees. Let your hips lower slightly. Stay in this position for three breaths.

Sun Salutation Pose

1. Stand with your feet together and your arms relaxed at your side. Pull your shoulders down and back.

2. While inhaling deeply, raise your arms overhead, reaching upward with your palms facing each other.

3. Then, as you exhale slowly, bend at the waist and gently push your hips back, so you fold forward. Only come down as far as is comfortable for your back; bend your knees if you need to.

4. Next, bring your right leg back into a lunge, dropping your right knee to the floor. Press both legs to the floor to keep your balance as you raise your arms up, inhaling.

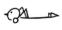

5. Exhale as you lower your arms, putting each hand on either side of your left foot and then bring that left foot back to meet your right foot; come to all fours.

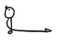

6. On the next inhalation, drop your chest down. Using your arm strength, bring your chin to the floor between your hands.

7. Slowly lift up your head and chest, being careful not to strain your neck. Keep your shoulders back and down and bring your shoulder blades together, feeling the nice opening this brings into your chest.

8. On the exhalation, use your arms and legs to press your hips back to rest as closely to your heels as possible. Take a few deep breaths here.

9. Next, come to all fours, with your hands directly under your shoulders and your knees directly under your hips. Slowly, straighten your arms and press your hips back into a teepee shape. Keep the weight off your shoulders by pressing your hips further back, bending your knees if necessary.

10. Lift your right leg forward to your hands, so you come into a lunge position. Inhale and bring your arms up, remembering to press down on your legs to keep your balance.

11. On the next exhalation, lower your hands to each side of your right foot, bring your left foot forward to meet the right, and come to a forward folded position.

12. Inhale as you lift up your torso, raising your arms overhead. Exhale, lower your arms to your sides, and come to a standing pose. You're done! A complete salutation to the sun. Do this every morning and it will make your day.

Tai chi

You've probably seen people practicing tai chi in movies or in parks around your city. Tai chi chuan is a martial arts form that is often performed slowly and gracefully. It looks like a very slow dance. Although it won't lower blood glucose levels, tai chi can improve your mood, provide relaxation through a meditative state, and build muscle fitness. You can learn tai chi from certified instructors or an instructional video or DVD.

PERSONAL GOAL

This week (date _____), I decided I can
(*check one*):

☐ Massage my neck and stretch my shoulders at work.
☐ Stretch when I see my cat or dog stretch.
☐ Incorporate yoga into my daily activities.
☐ Find out about local yoga or tai chi classes.
☐ Get the Yoga Fan from www.trainingfan.com or try out some YogaToes (a device that stretches and exercises your toes) from www.yogapro.com.
☐ Find a certified tai chi instructor or get a "Tai Chi for Diabetes" video from www.taichifordiabetes.com.
☐ Make time to meditate for five minutes.

 Will yoga take the knots out of my stomach?

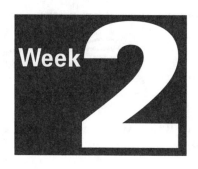

Week 2

Minute-by-Minute Glucose Monitoring

What is continuous glucose monitoring?

Ever thought it'd be awesome to know your blood glucose level minute by minute, hour after hour? Well, continuous glucose monitoring (CGM) is the answer. It's not perfect (you'll have to double check highs and lows using a traditional fingerstick test and most CGM devices require twice-a-day calibration by self-blood glucose monitoring), but it's pretty close. Imagine the self-management power you'll have if you are able to see exactly what your blood glucose level is just before eating a meal or right after exercise. These are the benefits that CGM offers.

How does CGM work?

CGM devices work by measuring the glucose concentration of your interstitial fluid (fluid that is just under the skin). A small needle is inserted under the skin with a tiny plastic tube (devices called "introducers" help you do this with relatively little pain). The needle is immediately removed and the plastic tube, also called the sensor, remains taped in position for up to three days. The nickel- or quarter-sized sensor is usually taped to your arm or abdomen and sends your blood glucose levels to the pager-sized monitor or receiver or, on some models, an insulin pump. CGM devices also have alarms to alert you when your blood glucose is going especially high or low.

Sounds nice, but I bet it's expensive.

Yes, *but* a trip to the emergency room, a loss of a day's work, or a disruption in your life spent treating and recovering from hypoglycemia is also quite costly. Transmitters and receivers vary in range from $800 to $2,000. Sensors (which are typically changed every three days) cost about $35 each. Insurance providers have been slow to pay for this new tool. If you think a CGM device sounds right for you, discuss it with your health care provider at your next appointment.

PERSONAL GOAL

This week (date _____), I decided I can (*check one*):

☐ Ask my diabetes educator about CGM.
☐ Go over the pros and cons of CGM with my physician.
☐ Ask if anyone in my diabetes support group is wearing one and if they'd share their experience.
☐ Visit the websites of these device manufacturers: DexCom (www.dexcom.com), Medtronic (www.minimed.com), and Abbott (www.freestylenavigator.com).
☐ Visit a diabetes blog to read what others are saying about CGM (consider the source, too).
☐ Ask myself if I am willing to go into high gear with learning about my diabetes.
☐ Ask my spouse or partner for support in learning about CGM.
☐ Other: _____.

CGM is like putting a leash on a wild dog, you'll get dragged along for a little while.

Over-the-Counter Drugs and Treatments

You can buy many types of medications and treatment remedies without a prescription, but how do you know which ones are safe with your diabetes and other conditions? For instance, some cold medicines may raise your blood glucose, and certain painkillers may raise blood pressure. So when it comes to over-the-counter (OTC) drugs and treatments, always check with your health care provider to see if it's okay.

Here are some tips to think about when buying OTC drugs.

- Check the label to know what you're getting. Choose sugar-free products. Search for warnings advising people with diabetes or high blood pressure against taking the medicine or using the product. For example, on wart removal products, you'll see a statement that reads, "Not to be used by people with diabetes."
- Acetaminophen-containing drugs (such as Tylenol) have a risk for severe liver damage *if* more than the maximum recommended dose is taken in 24 hours or if taken by people who have three or more alcoholic drinks in a day. In 2002, 26,000 people were hospitalized and 450 deaths were attributed to acetaminophen overdoses.
- Non-steroidal anti-inflammatory drugs (NSAIDs), such as ibuprofen (Advil), aspirin, naproxen (Aleve), and Ketoprofen, have a risk for stomach bleeding for people over age 60, who are taking a blood thinner or steroid, who have three or more alcoholic drinks a day, or who take it longer than directed.

Some Diabetes-Friendly OTC Drugs

Allergies
- Chlor-Trimeton
- Neo-Synephrine
- Claritin
- Loratadine

Antacids
- Alka-Seltzer
- Di-Gel
- Maalox
- Mylanta
- Prilosec
- Tums (sugar-free)
- Zantac

Anti-diarrhea
- Diasorb
- Immodium A-D
- Pepto-Bismol

Cold and cough
- Ayre nasal spray
- Diabetic Tussin
- Dimetapp
- Naldecon
- Robitussin (sugar-free)
- Safe-Tussin
- Simply Saline nasal spray
- Sugar-free cough drops/ throat sprays

Laxative
- Colace
- Citrucel
- Fiberall
- Metamucil (sugar-free)
- Phillips Milk of Magnesia
- Psyllium Husk Fiber (sugar-free)

Motion sickness
- Bonine
- Dramamine

Pain/fever relief
- Advil or Motrin (ibuprofen)
- Aleve (naproxen)
- Bayer aspirin (salicylate)

Vitamins
- Caltrate
- Flintstones
- Geritol
- One-A-Day

Millions of people take OTC medications. Complications are rare, but you can make your risks nonexistent by taking extra care in choosing safe products.

PERSONAL GOAL

This week (date _____), I decided I can (*check one*):

☐ Have a chat with my health care provider about OTC drugs and treatments that are safe to use.
☐ Bring my vitamins to my registered dietitian for analysis.
☐ Make sure my health care team knows all of the OTC drugs I take and bring a list of them to every appointment.
☐ Read medication and product labels.
☐ Select sugar-free and alcohol-free medications whenever possible.
☐ Other: _____.

 I have to buy a magnifying glass to read these warning labels.

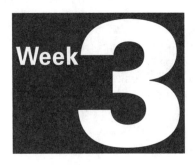

Week 3

The Hospital Twilight Zone

Being hospitalized for a planned or unplanned medical event is like stepping into a Twilight Zone episode—it's a new dimension and may be filled with surprises and interesting twists, especially if you let your diabetes guard down.

Ironically, when you're sick in a hospital bed you would think you'd get a break from being your diabetes project manager, but it sometimes doesn't work that way. Some hospitals do not have standardized methods for effectively managing and identifying hyperglycemia, so it's important to keep aware of your diabetes status. This does not apply to all hospitals, but like all things regarding diabetes, it's always better to be prepared.

Preparing for the Twilight Zone

You can take several steps to ensure that your hospital stay is as successful as possible.

- Find an advocate or be your own advocate. Ask a family member or friend to watch out for your health while in the hospital or request to see a diabetes educator who can help. Ask your doctor to order blood glucose tests before meals and at bedtime. Contact a diabetes specialist (you can request to see an endocrinologist or pick up the phone and call your own).
- Bring in your meter, supplies, and a complete medication list.
- For planned procedures, try to get the earliest time slot, so you can lower the risks of going low if you have to avoid eating before and/or after the procedure. Check with your health care provider about medication and insulin adjustments for the day of the procedure.

- Embrace insulin. Don't freak out if you need insulin during your hospital stay. It is often the best way to maintain good blood glucose levels while you're in the hospital.
- Wear medical identification (bracelet or necklace) in case of emergencies. This will help emergency staff know that you have diabetes.
- If you wear an insulin pump, call the hospital to find out if it is acceptable to keep using it during your stay.

PERSONAL GOAL

This week (date _____), I decided I can (*check one*):

- ☐ Request to be the first on the list for any procedures or surgery.
- ☐ Choose an advocate for my hospitalization.
- ☐ Bring my glucose monitor and supplies to the hospital.
- ☐ Ask if having a regular bedtime snack is appropriate.
- ☐ Ask what medications I am being given and why.
- ☐ Request to use my own lancets (with the hospital's glucose monitor) to decrease pain.
- ☐ Speak up and ask to speak to the charge nurse, a diabetes educator, or my endocrinologist if my blood glucose levels are not well controlled while I'm in the hospital.
- ☐ Other: _____.

**I used to be afraid of snakes.
Now I'm afraid of the hospital.**

Diabetes Dollars and Sense

 Let's be frank: diabetes self-care is expensive, and that can add a lot of stress to your daily life. The direct, inflation-adjusted cost of diabetes in the U.S. in 2007 was $116 billion. Indirect costs from disability, lost work, and premature death add another $58 billion to that total. People with diabetes pay a higher out-of-pocket cost for health care. Medical expenditures are higher for people with diabetes than for those without diabetes.

Saving your health and your health care bucks

Here are some tips on maximizing your health care dollars wherever you go.

At home

- Get friendly with your health insurance company. Find out exactly what is covered: from medications to test trips to co-pays for medical visits and diabetes classes.
- Look for coupons in diabetes magazines or incentives through diabetes supply manufacturers' literature and websites.
- Check for local programs that provide health care or supplies to individuals in need (the diabetes program or medical social worker at your local hospital will have the most knowledge about these resources).
- Take the time to research the programs from pharmaceutical companies that offer free drugs to people in need.
- Review your medical bills for accuracy, and don't be shy to ask for itemized explanations. You may catch expensive errors.

At the health care provider's office

- Frankly discuss the burden of out-of-pocket costs.
- Bring a list of medications covered by your insurance provider.
- Ask if you can switch to generic versions of any prescriptions.
- Ask if it's possible to have a higher dose of medication prescribed that can be cut in half (with a pill cutter, or some pharmacists will do this for you). This gives you twice the medicine for the same price. Not all pills can be cut, so this does not apply to all medications.

- Find out if your medications come in a combination form.
- Ask for samples of your medication or test strips.

At the pharmacy
- Shop around, especially for test strips, which tend to cost less at bigger chain pharmacies, such as Costco, Walgreen's, or Sam's Club.
- Ask if a 90-day supply of prescriptions would be less expensive.
- Request information about prescription assistance (programs that provide medications to people who cannot afford the out-of-pocket costs).

On the Internet
- Avoid scams. Watch out for fake products that promise you the moon. Before you spend one hard-earned cent on the web, check out the FDA website (www.fda.gov/buyonline). You'll be amazed at the number of people trying to lure you into buying bogus products.
- Check in with the Partnership for Prescription Assistance to find programs that provide free or nearly free medications (www.pparx.org).

At work
- Sign up for a flexible spending account that allows you to use pre-tax dollars for your health care costs. Check with your benefits coordinator for information about these wonderful programs.
- Before leaving a job, talk to the human resources staff about purchasing extended health insurance through the Consolidated Omnibus Budget Reconciliation Act (COBRA) or ask about other options.

What about Medicare and Medicaid?

Medicare is a federal program that provides health coverage for people over age 65, those who are disabled, and those with kidney failure. To learn more about Medicare benefits, call the National Diabetes Education Program at 1-800-438-5383 and ask for a copy of "The Power Is In Your Hands" and "Expanded Medicare Coverage of Diabetes Services."

Medicaid is a state government program that provides health insurance for qualified individuals in need. Programs differ among states. Check the local pages of your phonebook to get in contact with your local office.

What if don't have insurance?

If you don't have insurance, contact the Bureau of Primary Health Care, a service of the Health Resources and Service Administration, to find local health centers that offer health care regardless of your ability to pay by calling 1-800-400-2742 or visit their website at www.bphc.hrsa.gov.

PERSONAL GOAL

This week (date _____), I decided I can (*check one*):

☐ Discuss the costs of diabetes with my health care provider.

☐ Start a flexible spending account at work so I can use pre-tax dollars to pay for health care expenses.

☐ Check out the Partnership for Prescription Assistance at www.pparx.org or call 1-888-477-2669.

☐ Check out the Food and Drug Administration's website for tips on safely purchasing prescription medications online at www.fda.gov/buyonline and click on the "Warning Letters to Online Sellers" section.

☐ Make a plan to improve my financial health, work to pay off debts, and build up savings.

☐ Learn to be a savvy consumer by ordering the "Consumer Action Handbook" from the Federal Citizen Information Center by visiting www.ConsumerAction.org or calling 1-888-878-3256.

☐ Before buying something, ask myself if it will improve my life and move me closer to my goals.

☐ Other: _____.

Money might not be able to buy happiness, but it can sure buy a lot of test strips.

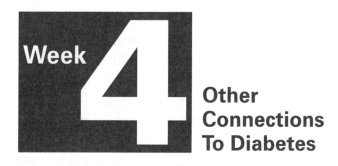

Week 4 — Other Connections To Diabetes

Diabetes has far-reaching effects on many other health issues. Here are a few notable issues listed alphabetically.

Alzheimer's disease (AD)
The higher your A1C level (especially when above 12%), the higher your risk for AD. Even people with pre-diabetes have a higher risk for AD.

Disaster planning
Keep a backpack full of all of the equipment you'd need for at least two weeks in a safe and secure location. Include a waterproof and insulated kit for testing supplies, medications, prescription numbers (especially handy if they are from national pharmacy chains and can be filled throughout the country), copies of recent lab tests, and other medical information. Mark your calendar so you know to check the expiration dates of these supplies every six months. During the aftermath of Hurricane Katrina, thousands of people with diabetes were stranded without medication and supplies for many days, resulting in medical emergencies.

Hearing loss
Diabetes is associated with hearing loss. When is the last time you had a hearing test or a comprehensive examination with an audiologist? What are you doing to prevent hearing loss? Think about that, and turn down the volume on the TV and your iPod and minimize your exposure to noisy environments.

Insulin allergies

One of every 200 insulin users may experience an allergic reaction to the additives in the insulin they inject. These additives and buffers help the insulin stay stable and prevent the growth of mold and bacteria. Allergic reactions are quite rare. They tend to appear as redness, itchiness, or hives that remain for several days around injection sites. Allergists can run tests to determine what is causing the reactions and treat your allergy with desensitization, a process that gradually reduces or eliminates a person's allergic reaction to insulin.

Women and lipid management

Women tend to have greater difficulty meeting healthy levels of LDL cholesterol, but they do have better success at meeting HDL cholesterol and triglyceride goals.

Women with diabetes skip mammogram screening.

Despite regular health care visits, women with diabetes are less likely to get a routine mammogram. It can be easy to put aside other health issues if you're always running to the doctor's office to tend to your diabetes, but mammograms are an important part of female health. Remember to pay attention the rest of your body.

PERSONAL GOAL

This week (date _____), I decided I can (*check one*):

☐ Pack an emergency/disaster supply kit in a back-pack or suitcase with wheels that has at least two weeks' worth of medication, glucose tablets, water (at least one gallon of water), test strips, an extra glucose meter, a large box of saltine crackers, a jar of peanut butter, a small box of powdered milk, dry cereal, packages of cheese and crackers, utensils, cans of tuna, nuts, socks, underwear, a sweatsuit, and a battery-operated radio.

☐ Request to see an allergist if I'm having a reaction at my insulin injection sites (redness, swelling, itching).

☐ Get my complete cholesterol panel done if I haven't in the past six months.

☐ Check my glucose before driving.

☐ Get my routine mammogram exam.

☐ Other: _____.

Invest in hearing aids— they'll replace all those iPod earphones one day.

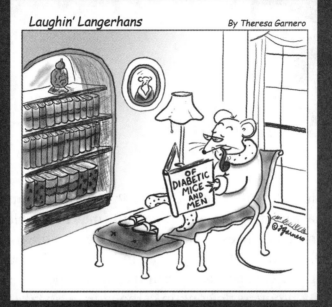

Laughin' Langerhans — By Theresa Garnero

Month 11

Week 1

Blue
Is for Milk

Blue is for milk because the MyPyramid spectrum doesn't have white. Granted, nonfat milk may have a bluish hue, and blue cheese and blueberry yogurt do exist. Before you think about this until you're blue in the face, pick out two of the following goals to approach the milk, yogurt, and cheese group. Milk and milk products do contain carbohydrate, so take this into account when you are making these food decisions.

PERSONAL GOAL

This week (date _____), I decided I can (*check one*):

☐ Ask that my latte or cappuccino be made with nonfat or low-fat milk.
☐ Try a nonfat cheese.
☐ Use nonfat or low-fat milk when making a creamy vegetable soup (like cream of mushroom or broccoli).
☐ Substitute low-fat yogurt in dishes where I'd normally use sour cream (e.g., enchiladas, baked potatoes).
☐ Make a fruit or veggie dip with yogurt.
☐ Try calcium-fortified juices, cereal, soy beverages, and bread.
☐ Get my calcium from soybeans, dark leafy greens, and canned fish.
☐ Other: _____.

Medication Literacy

What does literacy have to do with diabetes self-management? If you can read and understand health information, then you are more likely to take your medications correctly and have a better chance at controlling your diabetes. But there's more to it than that. Literacy is the key to successfully navigating medication adjustments, counting carbohydrates, and understanding how to respond to blood glucose levels. The more medications you take, the more likely you are to make mistakes (especially for those who take more than five medications). Insulin has so many variables that affect its dosage that it can be very easy to make mistakes.

Know Your Medications

Ask these questions whenever you receive a medication.
- What does this drug do?
- Why am I taking this drug?
- When do I take my pills?
- How many pills do I take?
- Do I take it with food or can I take it anytime?
- What should I do if I miss a dose?
- How long will I be taking this drug?
- Will this drug have any interactions with my other medications? Here's a list of what I currently take.
- What side effects should I know about and what do I do if I notice them?

When you go to the doctor and the pharmacist, bring along this list of questions. Ask every one of them and write down the answers. Now, you can refer to this piece of paper whenever you have a question about any of your medications.

Do you know what this wording means? "Take one tablet daily for seven days, then two tablets twice a day." For the first seven days that you take this medication, you take only one tablet a day. After day seven, you will take two pills at a time, two times a day, probably in the morning and evening. It's a short sentence, but there's a lot of important information there. If you misunderstand this information, the drugs may not work correctly; or worse, they could harm you.

A recent study reported that people who read at or below the sixth-grade level frequently misunderstand dosage information on pill bottles. Although most participants could recite what was on the label, more than 45% *did not understand* at least one of the instructions for dose, timing, or duration. Don't open yourself up to these simple, but dangerous, mistakes. When you receive a prescription, ask your health care provider and pharmacist many questions about how to take the drug.

PERSONAL GOAL

This week (date _____), I decided I can (*check one*):

☐ Put all of my medications in a bag and review them with my pharmacist or health care provider.
☐ Go through all my medication bottles and prescriptions and throw away any I'm not using or that have expired.
☐ Go over all of my medication names, doses, frequency, purposes, and side effects, including OTC drugs, vitamins, and herbal remedies. Make a chart with this information, so it is easily available.
☐ Be able to recognize my medications by shape, color, size, and name.
☐ Other: _____.

My mind is literally like an artificial pancreas and jumbo carb calculator.

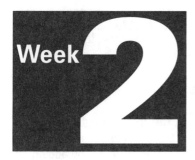

Week 2

The Good, the Bad, and the Ugly: Menopause and Testosterone

Diabetes aside, hormone imbalances are usually associated with women in menopause. However, men may also have hormone issues; specifically, they may have low testosterone. This section will help you understand the impact that menopause and low testosterone have on diabetes and your life.

	MENOPAUSE	LOW TESTOSTERONE
Description	When menstrual periods stop and ovaries start to shrivel, estrogen and progesterone production fade as well.	Low testosterone levels result from problems in the testes or with the hypothalamus (a small gland in the brain).
Age	Menopause begins around age 51, but can begin as early as 40 or earlier in women whose ovaries are surgically removed.	Low testosterone can begin around age 45 and older. It affects twice as many men with diabetes as the rest of the population, and only 10% of them get treatment.
Impact on blood glucose levels	May cause fluctuations, especially during perimenopause (the years leading up to menopause).	May raise blood glucose as a result of fatigue, sleep loss, and weight gain.
Symptoms	Menstrual period irregularity (with one to three cycles a year prior to stopping completely), hot flashes, sweating, irritability, insomnia, and vaginal dryness. Symptoms may continue for years.	Decreased strength and muscle mass, decreased bone density, low sex drive, erectile dysfunction, fatigue, and depression.
Shared diabetes symptoms	Lows: sweating and irritability. Highs: fatigue, mood swings, and vaginal dryness.	Sexual dysfunction, fatigue, and depression.
Weight	Risk of weight gain.	Overweight men are twice as likely to have low testosterone levels.

	MENOPAUSE	LOW TESTOSTERONE
Risks	Increased risk for osteoporosis; stress from lack of sleep may raise blood glucose levels.	Increased risk for falls.
Fertility	Fertility decreases after age 40, but conception is still possible.	Associated with low sperm count.
Treatment	<ul><li>Hormone replacement therapy (HRT) is a treatment that increases hormone levels in women experiencing menopause.</li><li>The Women's Health Initiative showed that HRT slightly increased the risks of breast cancer, stroke, and dementia.</li><li>HRT prevents osteoporosis.</li><li>Prescription vaginal estrogen (in cream, tablet, or ring formats) may help with pain and lubrication issues. OTC vaginal moisturizers are also available.</li></ul>	The primary method of treatment is to increase testosterone levels by adding more. This is achieved in a few ways:<ul><li>A tablet applied to the upper gums.</li><li>Gels that can be applied to the stomach or upper arms.</li><li>Patches that can be applied once a week.</li><li>Injections that are given about every two weeks.</li></ul>

PERSONAL GOAL

This week (date _____), I decided I can (*check one*):

☐ Consult with my health care team about the best approach to deal with my hormone issues.

☐ Contact the North American Menopause Society at 440-442-7550 or visit www.menopause.org for a free monthly newsletter.

☐ Ask to be tested for low testosterone and have the blood test in the morning, when levels are peaking.

☐ Report breast tenderness to my health care team.

☐ Report my decreased strength or height to my health care provider.

☐ Other: _____.

My glands have issues.

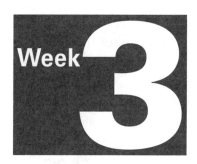

Week 3

Going the Extra Mile

This section is for those of you who are going the extra mile with an activity program or if you are a flat-out athlete. Even if you don't exercise (for whatever reason)—or are not planning on outdoing Gary Hall Jr.'s Olympic gold medal record—you can still pick up a pointer or two.

Exercise nutrition

When your body is at rest, it gets about 60% of its energy from fat and 40% from carbohydrates. During exercise, the body turns to carbohydrates for energy. The harder the workout and intensity, the more the body leans on carbs for fuel. This sounds reasonable, but where is that energy coming from? If you are exercising before or between meals, you may need a snack, especially if you plan on more than 30 minutes of activity.

As a review, consider having a snack before exercise to prevent hypoglycemia if your blood glucose is less than 100 mg/dl, you're going to exercise before a meal, you will be active for more than an hour, or your medication or insulin is peaking. Based on a 150-pound per-

Quick Snacks to Help Fuel My Body
- GU Energy Gel (it's maltodextrin and fructose) or GU Sports Drink (call 510-527-4664 or visit www.gusports.com to find out more).
- Sports drinks with up to 8% carbohydrate (higher percentages may cause cramping and diarrhea).
- Electrolytes for events over two hours in length (e.g., Gatorade).
- Don't forget water. You need it to prevent dehydration. Have some when you start to sweat. Go for room temperature water (cold water will go through your system faster).

son, you'd need about 30–40 grams of carbohydrate for one hour of moderate-intensity exercise or as much as 55 grams for high-intensity workouts. If you weigh more, you'll need more of a snack. In addition, the protein requirements for athletes dedicated to their sport are nearly double (about 100 grams a day). Remember to discuss exercise nutrition with a dietitian prior to becoming a full-time athlete.

How do I get my body ready for a several-hour event?

Eat a high-carb diet for about a week before the event, which is about 4 grams of carb per pound of body weight. For someone who weighs 150 pounds, that's 600 grams of carb a day. Make sure your medication can cover the added carbs so you won't be running on high blood glucose levels. Be sure to taper down your activity a couple of days before the big event. Your body needs a couple of days to rebuild nutrient stores and repair tissue. If you are trying to run a marathon, participate in a triathlon, or do something equally ambitious and you haven't seen your dietitian for an individualized nutrition plan, I will come and find you. That's flat-out dangerous. Make exercise nutrition a part of your training program.

Glucose Chutes and Ladders

Strenuous exercise can whip your blood glucose levels around like a birthday balloon in the wind. Let's review some key points.

- Hypoglycemia may occur during the exercise or be delayed into the next day. Frequently check your glucose before, during, and up to 24 hours after exercise. Carry your usual hypoglycemia treatment pack. The symptoms of a low may not be as obvious during exercise, which is why your life depends on regular glucose monitoring.
- Hyperglycemia may temporarily result from bursting-type or competitive sports, such as weightlifting, baseball, track, swimming, gymnastics, and figure skating. This is caused from a release of hormones that free stored glucose during exercise. After exercise, the sugar goes back into the bank (the liver), which is why lows can occur so many hours later. If your blood glucose stays high after exercise, you may need a slight medication adjustment.

Insulin deep thoughts

On the days you exercise hard, you will need a different plan for your insulin doses. Here are some basic principles, but remember to talk to your health care provider before you make changes.

Basal insulin. Unless you are planning to exercise for more than two hours, your long-acting insulin dose can stay the same. For more than two hours of activity, plan on reducing your basal dose by 20% (up to 30% for hardcore, several-hour events) for the day before the event. Be aware that weather can affect your blood glucose levels.

Bolus insulin. You may want to take 70% of your usual premeal insulin dose for 30–60 minutes of activity, 50% for one hour of heavy-duty exercise, or 35% for more than two hours of vigorous exercise.

Correction doses. Use half of what you normally would to cover your highs.

PERSONAL GOAL

This week (date _____), I decided I can (*check one*):

- ☐ Pay a visit to a registered dietitian who is also a certified diabetes educator and specializes in exercise (call the American Association of Diabetes Educators at 800-338-3633 and ask for help locating someone from the Physical Activity Specialty Practice Group).
- ☐ Talk to my health care provider about adjusting my medications to handle extra carbs during periods of extreme activity.
- ☐ Check my blood glucose every 30–60 minutes during vigorous exercise, more often if I feel strange.
- ☐ Carry my hypoglycemia treatment pack and ketone test strips.
- ☐ Other: _____.

Sugar Ray had to live up to his name.

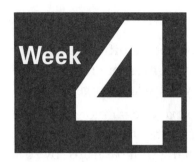

Week 4

Peace
If You Please

Time to keep the peace: the inner peace, that is. Reducing your stress levels is good for diabetes management. Choose from this list of stress-busting suggestions to soothe your mind and relax.

PERSONAL GOAL

This week (date _____), I decided I can (*check one*):

☐ Turn off the TV, close my eyes for five minutes, and let my thoughts drift.

☐ Buy a bouquet (or pick one from my garden) and marvel at the colors of nature.

☐ Be a source of love.

☐ Slow down a little bit to stay "in the moment."

☐ Call a friend who is upbeat.

☐ Pick up that book I've been meaning to read.

☐ Let go of something that I've been resenting.

☐ Other: _____.

I heard Karma means watching your body, mouth, and mind. You're fun to watch.

Anemia and Diabetes

 The connection between diabetes and anemia
Blood is composed of three main types of cells: white blood cells (fight infection), platelets (form clots in response to injury), and red blood cells (carry oxygen throughout the body and remove waste). Anemia is a condition in which the red blood cells have a reduced ability to carry oxygen throughout the body because of they lack a protein called hemoglobin or because the hemoglobin does not work as effectively as it used to. Moreover, red blood cells are produced in the kidneys, so if your diabetes affects your kidneys, then anemia may result. Anemia can also be caused by a lack of or low levels of iron.

How do I get tested for anemia?

If there is a chance that you have anemia, you will likely have to undergo a blood test called a complete blood count (CBC). The CBC measures your hemoglobin and hematocrit (percentage of red blood cells in blood). If you have low hemoglobin and hematocrit, you may be anemic.

A1C, anemia, and fructosamine

The A1C test measures the amount of glucose stuck to red blood cells. If you have anemia, A1C values become unreliable because there are fewer red blood cells to which glucose can attach itself. For

What are the signs of anemia?

- Feeling tired, weak, or fatigued
- Shortness of breath after very little activity
- Difficulty concentrating
- Frequent headaches
- Pale skin
- Rapid heartbeat
- Chest pain

Did you notice how several of these symptoms are similar to those of hypoglycemia? Take efforts to ensure that you don't have anemia instead of hypoglycemia.

people with diabetes and anemia, measuring fructosamine levels is the next best option.

Like A1C, your fructosamine level also represents your average blood glucose levels, but for only the previous two to three weeks. Fructosamine is formed when protein combines with glucose attached to the inside of a red blood cell. Measuring fructosamine is helpful for people with anemia and for people who have had rapid changes in their diabetes treatment (a new diet or medication) or are experiencing a pregnancy with diabetes.

There is no approved standardized rating for the results of a fructosamine test. If you have this test done, find out the ranges used by the lab, so you can correctly understand the test results.

How can I prevent anemia?

- Protect your kidneys by managing blood glucose and blood pressure levels.
- Get enough iron and vitamins in your diet.
- Avoid caffeine because it interferes with the absorption of iron.

How is anemia treated?

Iron supplements are the common treatment for most forms of anemia (there are many). Don't take iron unless you're told to because extra iron can be rough on your liver. Also, iron makes many people constipated. Some manufacturers solve this issue by combining iron with a stool softener. Your pharmacist can help you sort through iron options, if that's the route your health care provider suggests.

For other cases of anemia, there are many different forms of treatment. Some people need regular injections of erythropoietin to tell the kidneys to make more red blood cells. Others need injections of vitamin B12. For life-threatening anemia, people need blood transfusions.

PERSONAL GOAL

This week (date _____), I decided I can (*check one*):

☐ Report any of these symptoms to my health care provider: feelings of tiredness, weakness, or fatigue; shortness of breath; difficulty concentrating; frequent headaches; pale skin; rapid heartbeat; or chest pain.

☐ Get a CBC done or ask for my most recent CBC results (and look for the hemoglobin and hematocrit levels).

☐ Ask to have a fructosamine lab test if I've had a recent change in treatment or have anemia.

☐ Reduce my caffeine and/or alcohol intake.

☐ Learn more about anemia by contacting the National Anemia Action Council at 414-225-0138 or visiting www.anemia.org.

Maybe I'm anemic because diabetes causes me to have several irons in the fire.

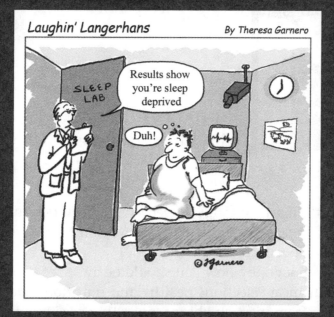

Month 12

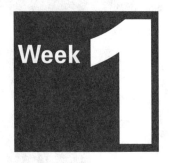

Week 1

Purple Is for
Meat and Beans

 It's time to test the U.S. Department of Agriculture for colorblindness. Purple meat? Maybe on Mars. Maybe they ran out of colors!

Seriously, though, by now you should be aware of the basics in keeping your meat selections healthy and nutritious. Our bodies need protein from meat and beans (and other vegetarian sources), but we just don't need a ton of it. So remember to keep trimming the fat from your meats and choosing healthy cooking methods, such as broiling and roasting over frying. Don't forget go always go lean. Make it your mantra.

You'll also notice that this part of the pyramid is relatively small. That's because meat and beans should compose a much smaller portion of your daily dietary intake than they do for most Americans.

In a nutshell

The rich and delicious flavor of nuts can be used to replace meat and beans in your diet. This is a simple, tasty, and healthy option that few people use to their advantage. Nuts can be an excellent source of unsaturated fats and protein. When buying nuts, select ones that are fresh and unsalted. Store nuts in an air-tight container (they can last up to six months in the refrigerator and up to a year in the freezer).

PERSONAL GOAL

This week (date _____), I decided I can (*check one*):

☐ Avoid chicken, turkey, and pork products that are labeled as "self-basting" (meaning a salt-containing solution has been added).

☐ Limit liver and other organ meats, as they are high in cholesterol.

☐ Choose fish rich in omega-3 fatty acids more often (e.g., salmon and trout).

☐ Add more vitamin E to my life by choosing sunflower seeds, almonds, or hazelnuts.

☐ Lean toward the lean (with round steaks, round roasts, top loin, top sirloin, tenderloin, pork loin, ham, at least 90% lean ground beef, and skinless chicken).

☐ Hide from breaded and fried dishes.

☐ Spread hummus on warm pita bread.

☐ Experiment with some vegetarian options, such as tofu.

☐ Toss some chickpeas, kidney beans, and pecans on a green salad instead of meat or cheese.

☐ Add toasted almonds, peanuts, or cashews to a veggie stir-fry instead of meat.

☐ Other: _____.

Butter is a discretionary calorie. I never was discreet.

Ready, Set, and...Stop?

 Are you having a difficult time sticking with an exercise program? Nearly half of people who start an activity regimen stop within six months. For many people, a great motivator is to join a gym or health club. Some people swear by them, others just swear. If anything, the fees for the gym will be a great motivator to get your money's worth out of the relationship.

Gyms and Health Clubs: Tips for the Savvy Shopper

1. *Convenience.* Studies have shown that if the gym is more than 12 minutes away, people tend to stop going. Make sure that your gym is close and convenient.
2. *Timing.* Check if the hours of operation fit into your schedule and stop by to see how busy it is when you'll be going. Peak times are typically 4–7 p.m. You need to know if there will be enough equipment available.
3. *Equipment.* Look around to see if there is a wide variety of well-maintained machines. If you see dust bunnies and built-up grime, go elsewhere.
4. *Personal trainers and class variety.* Ask about classes and the availability of fitness professionals who can get you started with an individualized program.
5. *Trial memberships.* Most gyms offer a free daily or weekly pass. Give it a test drive. Do you like the environment? Does it make you want to return?
6. *Get recommendations.* Ask people who attend the gym what they like and dislike.
7. *Expense.* Ask what's included in your contract or if there are hidden fees (sometimes towels and lockers cost extra). Ask about special offers or if the gym is part of a chain, so you can go to different locations. Ask whether their policy allows you to suspend your membership for illness and vacation and whether penalties apply if you cancel your membership.

PERSONAL GOAL

This week (date _____), I decided I can (*check one*):

- ☐ Ponder what it will take to become active the rest of my life.
- ☐ Ask friends, family members, and coworkers about which gyms they attend.
- ☐ Research some local gyms and visit a few.
- ☐ See if there are free gym opportunities in my local community or workplace.
- ☐ Ask my benefits coordinator at work if my employer offers a gym benefit to help pay for memberships.
- ☐ Other: _____.

My active voice works out every day. Now I need to get my body into the action.

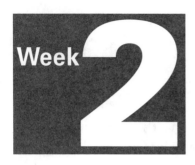

Week 2

While You Weren't Sleeping

Calling it a day? Maybe not. We live in a world where a good night's sleep seems to be on the verge of extinction. Shortchanging your sleep causes more than a droopy-eyed look of confusion and midday yawn-a-thons—it may raise blood glucose levels, cause other medical issues, and shorten your life.

Why is sleep important?

Every organ depends on adequate sleep to function properly. Sleep is a dynamic, complex activity. Signals sent out from the brain's command center, the hypothalamus, tell the body when to sleep,

What Is Sleep Apnea?

Sleep apnea is a sleeping disorder in which you stop breathing for extended periods. Sleep apnea is dangerous; it can increase night-time blood glucose levels and blood pressure and increases your risk for stroke, cardiovascular disease, and death. Signs you might have sleep apnea are loud snoring (although snoring doesn't always mean sleep apnea), headaches, dry mouth, feeling exhausted upon awakening, and sleeping at inappropriate times during the day (e.g., during work and driving). It's more common in men and in people who are overweight, smoke, or drink too much alcohol. A sleep specialist can diagnose the problem through physical exams or a trip to a sleep clinic. There are several treatment options for sleep apnea, including using a continuous positive airway pressure (CPAP) device (it pumps air through a special mask to keep the airway open, so breathing can continue during sleep) and some surgical procedures. Dental appliances are also available to help keep the tongue from falling to the back of the throat and blocking the airway during sleep.

wake up, adjust temperature, change blood pressure, help the immune system, and regulate hormones for digestion.

Did someone say digestion? If you're thinking about insulin, you're right on. Lack of sleep interferes with your ability to produce insulin. Lack of sleep interferes with your immunity to illness, which can make diabetes management problematic. Too little sleep also increases your risk for high blood pressure, depression, heart attacks, and strokes, which is even worse for your diabetes. If that's not bad enough, restless, sleepless nights increase the level of stress hormones in your body, causing the body to store fat and make it more difficult to lose weight.

How can I get more sleep?

Sleep hygiene. The bed is meant for sleep and sex, and if you're missing one, check out this list for sleep hygiene recommendations.

- Put yourself on a timeout to wind down for 30 minutes before bed.
- Get a new mattress and/or pillow.
- Try to go to bed and wake up around the same time every day.
- Avoid exercise and eating right before bed.
- Avoid caffeine (coffee or drinks) after lunch.
- Limit liquids after dinner.
- Limit alcohol intake.
- Don't eat or watch TV in bed.
- Try relaxing breathing exercises when you get into bed.
- After an *estimated* 20–30 minutes of not falling asleep, get out of bed (and don't obsessively watch the clock or it can stress you out and wake you up). Then, do something relaxing, like listening to music or reading something light, until you are sleepy enough to return to bed. Don't set up camp on the couch or you'll begin to associate sleep with the couch and not your bed.
- Talk to your health care provider.

Medications. Less than 10% of people with sleep disturbances take medication for the condition. Newer drugs include Rozerem (ramelteon), Lunesta (eszopiclone), and Ambien (zolpidem). They are quick acting and stay in the body for shorter periods than previous medications to aid in sleeping. If you need help sleeping, these can dramatically improve your quality of life. Be careful to report any weird symptoms; after taking sleeping pills for more than a few weeks, rare side effects may occur.

PERSONAL GOAL

This week (date _____), I decided I can (*check one*):

☐ Write down my worries and to-do list before my head hits the pillow, so I'm not dwelling on them while I try to sleep.

☐ Turn down the lights in my bedroom (e.g., wear an eyeshade or blackout shades, use clips to hold curtains in place, use 45-watt light bulbs in the bedroom, place low-wattage nightlights in hallways and bathrooms).

☐ Within an hour of waking, either go outside or go to a part of my home that gets a lot of light, so sunlight naturally wakes me up.

☐ Reduce clutter.

☐ Set the thermostat to 68–72°F.

☐ Avoid stimulating activities before bed or anything that can be upsetting (e.g., news, bills, hot topics with my spouse).

☐ Try the sleep hygiene tips above and talk to my health care provider about improving my sleep.

☐ Note how many hours of sleep I got in my blood glucose logbook to see if there is a correlation between my sleep patterns and blood glucose management.

☐ Search for a sleep center (a place where a specialist can examine my sleep patterns) in my area by visiting www.sleepcenters.org.

☐ Other: _____.

 I tried counting sheep. They ran off thinking I was a zombie.

What's the Alternative?

 Have you thought about trying complementary or alternative medical treatments? Maybe you're not familiar with this term. The most commonly used forms of complementary and alternative medicine are chiropractic care, herbal remedies, and relaxation techniques. Look at the list of other types of complementary and alternative medicine. Do you try any of these to help improve your diabetes self-care? You may realize that you've been following an "alternative" lifestyle all along.

Forms of Complementary and Alternative Medicine

- acupuncture
- Ayurveda
- biofeedback
- chelation
- chiropractic
- energy healing
- herbal remedies and supplements
- homeopathy
- hypnosis
- massage
- naturopathy
- Reiki therapy

A lot of people with diabetes use some of these therapies to help treat their diabetes. However, there is a lot of debate regarding their effectiveness and safety. Be sure to mention any complementary or alternative therapies to your health care team, so they can advise you about potential safety issues and make sure that you are, as always, not putting yourself at risk for further complications.

What about dietary supplements?

Dietary supplements can range from a daily multivitamin to fish oil pills, but the reason a person takes them is always the same: improved health. Regardless of which ones you take or are interested in taking, you should consult a registered dietitian about their safety, especially when combined with diabetes. Be sure to regularly monitor your blood glucose to make sure that supplements are not negatively affecting them. Take a look at some of the most common dietary supplements on the following page.

Type	Possible Effects	Considerations
Alpha-lipoic acid	Increases insulin sensitivity	Can cause nausea, vomiting, vertigo, and skin allergies.
Chromium picolinate	Improves insulin effectiveness	May pose an increased risk of hypoglycemia and renal problems.
Cinnamon	Increases insulin sensitivity	May cause hypoglycemia when combined with other diabetes drugs.
Fenugreek	Improves blood glucose levels	Don't use during pregnancy due to miscarriage risk.
Garlic	Improves blood glucose levels; increases insulin production and glucose storage in the liver	Has anti-clotting effects and may decrease the effectiveness of other drugs.
Ginseng (American or Asian types)	Improves blood glucose levels	May increase blood pressure and cause insomnia.
Gymnema	Improves blood glucose levels	May cause hypoglycemia.
Magnesium	Improves insulin sensitivity and action	May cause diarrhea; avoid if you have kidney problems.
Nopal (prickly pear)	Improves blood glucose levels and insulin sensitivity	May cause diarrhea or nausea.
Omega-3 fatty acids (fish oil)	Improves triglycerides; decreases risk for stroke and heart attack	May increase blood glucose levels.
Policosanol	Improves cholesterol levels	Use cautiously with anti-clotting medications (like aspirin).
Psyllium	Slows absorption of glucose and fat	Reduces absorption of other drugs; risk of hypoglycemia.
Vitamins (multivitamin)	Available in capsule, liquid, and tablet (including chewable) forms, multivitamins can help maintain a healthy body. Don't break the bank buying expensive vitamins. Your body will only absorb what it needs.*	

*Keep in mind that many people with diabetes do not get enough vitamin D. You may need to take more vitamin D than a multivitamin offers.

Better safe than sorry

Know what you're putting in your body. Supplement manufacturers are not regulated in the same fashion as drug companies, and they don't even have to register their products. Look for the USP label on supplements; it guarantees the integrity (content and dosage) of the supplement. Supplements aren't substitutes for healthy eating and being active.

PERSONAL GOAL

This week (date _____), I decided I can (*check one*):

☐ Consult a health practitioner trained in the use of supplements (e.g., a registered dietitian, pharmacist, or naturopath).

☐ Tell my health care team about all the supplements I'm taking.

☐ Try one supplement at a time, so I can figure out how each affects me.

☐ Take one multivitamin with breakfast.

☐ Stay away from scam products that say that you can permanently lose weight without exercising or that block the absorption of fat or carbohydrates.

☐ Visit the National Center for Complementary and Alternative Medicine of the National Institutes of Health (a free resource that provides referenced clinical information) at www.nccam.nih.gov/health/supplements.htm.

☐ Check out the National Institutes of Health Office of Dietary Supplements at http://ods.od.nih.gov/index.aspx.

☐ Other: _____.

 Can I use those herbal supplements as salad garnish?

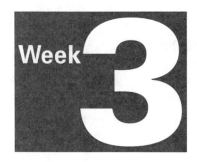

Week 3

Sequence for Success

You can monitor your own diabetes track record by using this form. It's in your best interest to keep an eye on the bigger diabetes picture. Work with your diabetes care team to cover each of these standards of care. Find a provider who matches or understands your style of communication.

Every Visit	Date ___	Date ___	Date ___	Date ___	Goals* or notes
Blood pressure					Below 130/80 mmHg
Weight					
Glucose review					Before meals 70–130 mg/dl; 2 hours after meals <180 mg/dl
Medication review					
Meal review					
Activity review					
Foot inspection					

Every Visit	Date ____	Date ____	Date ____	Date ____	Goals* or notes
Voice your concerns					

Every 3–6 Months	Date ____	Date ____	Date ____	Date ____	Goals*
A1C					Below 7%

Every 6 Months	Date ____		Date ____		Goals*
Dentist					Cleaning and checkup
Check disaster kit					Renew and replenish

Yearly	Date(s) _____	Goals* or notes
Physical exam		
Complete cholesterol panel		HDL: >40 mg/dl for men >50 for women LDL: <100 mg/dl (<70 is best) Triglycerides: <150 mg/dl (<100 is best)
Diabetes educator		
Eye exam		
Foot exam		
Flu shot		
Microalbumin		<30 mg/g (kidney test)
Ask about the pneumonia vaccine, aspirin use, and a thyroid checkup.		

*Goals are those suggested by the American Diabetes Association. Your health care provider may recommend different goals and frequency of tests and visits.

Tips for Health Care Visits

Be prepared for your visits by following these tips.
- Prepare a list of questions you want answered.
- Bring your blood glucose logbook (best if you bring a printout or photocopied form).
- Provide a list of all medications, their doses, and any herbal supplements you're taking.
- Complete a two- or three-day food diary to share during your visit.

During the visit
- Bring something in case you have to wait (e.g., a book or crossword puzzle).
- Bring along a friend or relative to help you remember all that was said and done.
- Be honest!
- Ask for printed materials or written instructions.

After the visit
- Call if you need clarification about anything.
- Follow through with your health care provider's instructions.

You are the most important person of the diabetes care team. Take an active role in your health to maximize the quality of care you receive.

PERSONAL GOAL

This week (date _____), I decided I can (*check one*):

☐ Take the extra step to make sure that I'm getting all of the tests that I need every year.

☐ Bring the chart to my appointments and ask them to enter my results.

☐ Ask my health care provider to conduct tests and evaluations that he or she may have forgotten.

☐ Be prepared for health care visits.

☐ Other: _____.

Diabetes Burnout

Not many people seem to like to talk about it, but there is an ugly side of diabetes that can come from being burned out on self-care. How are you feeling about having diabetes about now? Are you keeping up or fed up with self-care? Diabetes burnout is a common phenomenon when dealing with the never-ending demands of managing diabetes.

Do you ever feel...

- Aggravated?
- Angry?
- Like you explode easily at seemingly unimportant things?
- Beat up by diabetes?
- Bothered by everything related to your diabetes?
- Deprived of your favorite foods?
- Like no one understands your struggle?
- Negative and irritable?
- Overwhelmed?
- Exhausted?
- Hopeless?
- Isolated?
- Like there is a lack of support from those closest to you?

Have you stopped regularly checking your blood glucose, missed medical appointments, skipped refilling a prescription, or reverted to your old ways of eating that weren't in the best interest of your health? All of these are common, including the feelings described above, and indicate that you may be experiencing diabetes burnout.

Although diabetes burnout is common, it is also dangerous. Sometimes dealing with diabetes can make it feel like you're carrying the entire world on your shoulders, but the world doesn't want to be carried. It can be a huge burden when your blood glucose levels don't seem to want to work with you, but that isn't reason enough to quit checking your levels or doing the best you can to keep them under control. If diabetes burnout completely takes over, people stop checking their blood glucose, stop eating healthily, stop exercising, and stop taking their medications. Do you see anything wrong with this? Diabetes burnout puts people at greater risk of future complications and big problems in the present, like severe highs and lows.

If you're feeling discouraged or overwhelmed, seek out help from your health care team and support team right away. Definitely try to laugh; it can do wonders for your motivation level. Be sure to start small. Remember that you're not the only person who has ever felt down about diabetes, so there's no shame or fear in bringing this up with your support sources.

Dodging the Blood Sugar Police

A support group that is less than supportive can only make it worse. Do your family and friends help or hinder your efforts? Statements like the following don't help you or anyone else with diabetes:

- "You really shouldn't eat that." (But he or she keeps sweets in the house.)
- "You seem mad. Is your blood sugar high again?"
- "Why can't you just get your blood sugar under control?"
- "Why don't you exercise and lose weight?" (But he or she won't join you for a walk or any activity.)
- "Your doctor's not going to be happy with you." (But he or she brings home foods that aren't going to help your diabetes.)

If you feel like you're support group is not so supportive, you need to speak up. Point out that by being the blood sugar police, they're not helping you. Tell them that you're doing your best and that you need a cheerleader in your corner, not a traffic cop writing you tickets every time you slip up. Indicate that you appreciate help with your diet, but that it's not right to tempt you or encourage you to eat foods that are off your meal plan. If gentle discussions with your family and friends don't help, consider discussing your situation with your health care team. This isn't just about the people in your support group not helping you; it's about *you* and *your health*.

PERSONAL GOAL

This week (date _____), I decided I can (*check one*):

☐ Say "no" to things that don't support my goals, including people.
☐ Identify and acknowledge moments when I'm in denial.
☐ Identify what's stressing me out.
☐ Get my diabetes care team involved if I think I'm in diabetes burnout.
☐ Strive for my best and avoid perfectionism.
☐ Work on a hobby.
☐ Read a poem, look at art, or feed the birds.
☐ Other: _____.

Have a plan B, plan C, and plan Hawaii!

Week 4

Panorama Point

 Things don't always happen as planned, yet they have a way of working out. Getting diagnosed with diabetes may have been quite a shock and sent your life in a new direction. You may long for the life you had before getting diagnosed with diabetes, but you are still the same person, only wiser and potentially healthier because you've invested in your mental and physical well-being.

As with any crisis, your diabetes diagnosis has presented you with an opportunity to reflect and regroup. Looking back, what do you see from this vantage point? What have you learned about diabetes, yourself, and those around you? What strengths and vulnerabilities have you discovered?

Before we part, let's take some time to review your journey so far. This is not the end. It's the beginning. Another chapter in your life is about to begin. Remember to be strong and resourceful as you continue on. Even with diabetes, life can still have passion—so enjoy yourself. And always remember to laugh.

YEAR IN REVIEW

Today's date: _____

Look back over this past year and review the goals you made for yourself, focusing on one key decision at a time. Next to each area below, jot down at least one successful change you've made and one area that could use attention.

Keys to Success	Successful Change	Needs Attention
Eat wisely		
Be active		
Check numbers		
Reduce stress		
Understand medications		
Avoid problems		
Reduce risks		
Add humor		

Having some trouble?

Here are some things to think about as you fill out the chart above.

- On average, are my blood glucose levels 70–130 mg/dl before meals and less than 180 mg/dl two hours after meals?
- Can I sometimes identify why my blood glucose levels fluctuate?
- Was my last A1C less than 7%?
- Is my blood pressure less than 130/80 mmHg?
- Is my LDL cholesterol less than 100 mg/dl?
- Is my diet diabetes-friendly?
- Am I getting regular physical activity?
- Have I forgotten to take my medication this past week?
- Do I sabotage or rescue myself?
- Have I laughed at myself lately?
- Are my thoughts more positive than negative?
- What is working? What is not?
- Do I plan ahead to deal with potential problems?
- Am I willing to ask for help?
- Do I report when I have chest pain or pressure, dizziness or lightheadedness, difficulty breathing, balance problems, nausea, or muscle aches that last for days (warning signs of other problems)?
- Have I replaced my toothbrush recently?

PERSONAL GOAL

Thumb through this book on a regular basis so you can choose new goals or revisit ones you've already selected. In addition, here are some new ideas.

This year, I've decided that I can (*check two*):

☐ Go to a spa.
☐ Decide what I am not going to eat today or move to the skinniest state in the nation: Colorado (lots of opportunities for exercise).
☐ Change the tone of my internal voice.
☐ Find an activity that I love to do.
☐ Embrace slow, lasting weight loss by focusing on getting strong and healthy.
☐ Attend an intensive diabetes program.
☐ Research and investigate the latest in diabetes breakthroughs.
☐ Participate in a diabetes study, so I can help improve the status for all people with diabetes.
☐ Get involved with or volunteer for a diabetes organization in my community.
☐ Have the confidence to imagine reaching my goals.
☐ Pick up this book every week to pick out something new.
☐ Laugh always.

Happy trails to you, until we meet again.

Index

J

Joslin Diabetes Center, 158
Joslin Diabetes Center Exercise
Physiology Department, 222
Juvenile Diabetes Research
Foundation International
(JDRF), 158

K

*Keep Moving!....Keep Healthy with
Diabetes* (Joslin Diabetes
Center Exercise Physiology
Department), 222
ketoacidosis, 210–211
ketones, 211–212. *See also* diabetic
ketoacidosis (DKA)
kidneys, 95–97, 133, 275–277

L

labyrinth, 193
laxative, 255
LDL cholesterol, 86
Liberty Medical, 241
lipid levels, 86, 262–263
literacy, 267–268
liver problems, 68, 112

M

macrosomia, 9
mammogram screening, 262–263
management, key to, 2
marijuana, 232
meal planning, 12–15, 29–30,
143–144
meat, 280–281
Medicaid, 259–260
MedicAlert, 159
Medicare, 259–260
medication. *See also* insulin
alternative, 287–289

blood pressure, 127–129
cholesterol, 149–151
cost, 258–260
diabetic neuropathy, 225–226
dipeptidyl peptidase-4 (DPP-4)
inhibitors, 213–214
effectiveness, 108
facts about, 22–23
Glucophage (metformin), 68–69
hospitalization, 256–257
insulin secretagogue, 90–91
literacy, 267–268
mail order, 241
oral, 46–47
sick-day plan, 73
side effects, 45–48
sleep, 285–286
thiazolidinediones (TZDs), 47,
111–112
travel and, 134
Medicool, Inc., 241
meditation, 247
Medlineplus.com, 159
menopause, 132, 269–270
menstrual cycles, 132
Mental Health Association, 77
meter, blood testing, 125–126.
See also equipment; supplies
metformin, 68–69
microalbumin test, 96–97
milk, 120–121, 266
mind matters, 4–5, 242–243, 274
monochromatic infrared therapy
(Anodyne therapy), 225–226
monounsaturated fats, 81
moods, 75–77
motion sickness, 255
muscles, 187
MyPyramid, 159
myocardial infarction (MI),
154–156

R

relaxation techniques, 287
renin-angiotensin-aldosterone system (RAAS), 129
resistance training, 207–209
resources, 156–160
retinopathy, 152–153, 215
rivers, 230
Rule of 15, 39

S

salt, 184–185
saturated fats, 81
self-monitoring of blood glucose (SMBG), 18–21, 39–41, 57, 66–67, 125, 170–171, 252–253. *See also* glucose; hyperglycemia; hypoglycemia
serving sizes, 31–36, 57–58, 105. *See also* food; food pyramid; nutrition
sexual health, 130–133
sickness, 72–74, 180–182, 194–195
side effects, 45–48
site testing, 170–171
skin/skin care, 238–239
sleep, 284–286
sleep apnea, 155, 284
smoking, 92–94, 155, 232
socks, 113–114
sodium, 31
Somogyi effect, 108–109
spices, 185–186
spirituality, 193
statins, 149
steroids, 108
stress, 52–53, 108, 131, 155, 180–182, 274. *See also* illness
stroke, 154–156

supplements, 120–121
supplies, 241. *See also* equipment
support system, 24–25, 137–138, 156–160, 193. *See also* health care team
swimming pools, 230
symbols, 2
Symlin, 235–236
symptoms
    diabetic ketoacidosis (DKA), 211
    hyperglycemia, 40
    hyperglycemic hyperosmolar nonketotic syndrome (HHNS), 210
    hypoglycemia, 39
    neuropathy, 224
    periodontal disease, 70
syringe, 190–192

T

tai chi, 251
tea, 92
television resources, 156
testosterone, 269–270
thiazolidinediones (TZDs), 47, 111–112
thrush, 71
tobacco, 92–94, 155, 232
tonometry, 152
tooth care, 70–71, 155, 240
Training Fan, 167
trans fats, 81
transcutaneous electrical nerve stimulation (TENS), 225
travel, 134–136
treatment plan, 5, 132
triglycerides, 86
type 1 diabetes, 8–9
type 2 diabetes, 8–9

U

urinary tract infections (UTI),
132–133
urine test, 96–97

V

vacation, 134–136
vaginal yeast, 132
vegetables, 105–106, 218–219
vegetarian diet, 164–165
vial, 190

vision, 151–153, 215–216
visual acuity test, 151
vitamins, 255, 287–289

W

water activities, 230–231
weight, 12, 88–89, 140–144, 173

Y

year in review, 297–299
yoga, 247–251

Other Titles from the American Diabetes Association

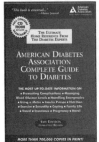

American Diabetes Association
Complete Guide to Diabetes, 4th Edition
by American Diabetes Association

Have all the tips and information on diabetes that you need close at hand. The world's largest collection of diabetes self-care tips, techniques, and tricks for solving diabetes-related problems is back in its fourth edition, and it's bigger and better than ever before.

Order no. 4809-04; NEW LOW PRICE! $19.95

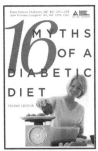

16 Myths of a Diabetic Diet, 2nd Edition
by Karen Hanson Chalmers, MS, RD, LDN, CDE, and Amy Peterson Campbell, MS, RD, LDN, CDE

16 Myths of a Diabetic Diet will tell you the truth about diabetes and how to eat when you have diabetes. Learn what the most common myths about diabetes meal plans are, where they came from, and how to overcome them. Diabetes doesn't have to be a life sentence of boring, dull meals. Let experts Karen Chalmers and Amy Campbell show you how to create and follow a healthy, enjoyable way of eating.

Order no. 4829-02; Price $14.95

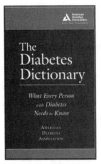

The Diabetes Dictionary
by American Diabetes Association

Diabetes can be a complicated disease; so to stay healthy, you need to understand the constantly growing vocabulary of diabetes research and treatment. *The Diabetes Dictionary* gives you the straightforward definitions of diabetes terms and concepts that you need to successfully manage your disease. With more than 500 entries, this pocket-size book is an indispensable resource for every person with diabetes.

Order no. 5020-01; Price $5.95

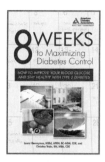

8 Weeks to Maximizing Diabetes Control

by Laura Hieronymus, MSEd, APRN, BC-ADM, CDE, and Christine Tobin, RN, MBA, CDE

In just 8 weeks, you can learn the tricks of the trade for managing your type 2 diabetes. Whether you've just been diagnosed or have been living with it for years, *8 Weeks to Maximizing Diabetes Control* gives you the tools and resources you need to reach your treatment goals.

Order no. 5017-01; Price $16.95

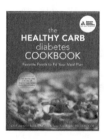

The Healthy Carb Diabetes Cookbook

by Lara Rondinelli, RD, LDN, CDE, and Chef Jennifer Bucko, MCFE

Worried about carbs? The 199 delicious recipes featured in *The Healthy Carb Diabetes Cookbook* prove that carbs aren't just okay—they're essential. Carefully constructed to be healthy and great tasting, each recipe in this book is handcrafted by Chef Jennifer Bucko and Lara Rondinelli, the team that brought people with diabetes the bestselling *Healthy Calendar Diabetic Cooking.*

Order no. 4666-01; Price $18.95

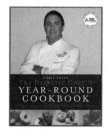

The Diabetic Chef's Year-Round Cookbook

by Chris Smith, The Diabetic Chef

Tired of uninspired, bland meals? Treat yourself to the Diabetic Chef's handcrafted recipes and bring market-fresh foods to your dining table. It doesn't matter whether you're preparing hors d'oeuvres for a small gathering or a weeknight dinner—you'll find whatever you need in *The Diabetic Chef's Year-Round Cookbook.*

Order no. 4667-01; Price $19.95

To order these and other great American Diabetes Association titles, call **1-800-232-6733** or visit **http://store.diabetes.org**. American Diabetes Association titles are also available in bookstores nationwide.